Kristy Cameron

Mitchell's Gift

**A parent's perspective on surviving life…
with a premature baby
in the NICU.**

By Kristy Cameron

This book is dedicated to my husband John.

* * * *

Because of your strong shoulders I was able to write this book. I love you.

A special thank you to my editor and friend, Elissa.

* * * *

You have worked miracles.

Contents

Forward

This book is for all the parents who suddenly find themselves thrown into the life of the Neo-natal Intensive Care Unit, or NICU. When I went through the experience of having a micro-preemie (Mitchell was born at 24 weeks), I desperately wanted to find a book about how parents felt during their time in the NICU. After finding only textbooks with clinical perspectives on the preemie and NICU experience, I vowed that this book would be written. I hope the following pages will help you cope with the incredible challenge of having a baby in the NICU.

Much love,

Kristy

1. The birth itself

The Joy of Pregnancy

When expecting a baby, we all dream of the day that we will have a cuddly bundle of joy in our arms.

What we're not ready for is our child's sudden and premature entry into the world -- an entry rife with possible complications.

Suddenly we find ourselves in a foreign part of the hospital where we never expected to be -- the NICU -- praying minute by minute for the health and survival of our baby.

The Shock of Delivery

I will always remember the moment I knew something was wrong. A mother's intuition is very powerful and she is attuned to every change that is happening within her body. I remember exactly where I was when the realization set in, what I said in the ambulance on the way to the hospital, and the moment I knew that life would never be the same. I'm sure you do, too.

It was about 4:00 a.m. when I was awakened by my water breaking, 24 weeks into my pregnancy. My husband and I threw on our clothes and were at the hospital moments later. The expressions on the doctors' and nurses' faces made me realize what a serious situation we were in. Until that moment, I'd been doing everything in my power to rationalize what was happening. The sympathetic looks from the hospital staff slapped me back to reality.

I was immediately placed in an ambulance and taken to a Level 3 Neonatal Intensive Care Unit where my baby would have a better chance of survival.

During the next several weeks, many events unfolded. It is likely that you will identify with certain aspects of my own experience and not with others. Each of our stories is unique, with its own twists and turns.

Over the next four days, the doctors administered several drugs in an attempt to alleviate the contractions. The most powerful drug was magnesium, which was so incapacitating that a nurse and my husband had to turn me from side to side whenever I wanted to move. I didn't have any muscle control and my body was tipped head down at what felt like an extreme angle.

On day four, despite the medications, my contractions started again. At this point, we were faced with an agonizing decision. We could wait and hope for more time, which would increase the risk of delivering Mitchell in a crisis situation, where he would have a lesser chance of survival. Our other option was to deliver him in a controlled environment where he would receive the best medical care available, but still be at risk of not surviving due to his young gestational age. What a choice! This wasn't how it was supposed to be. Mitchell was supposed to emerge a healthy robust baby in January of 2005, not a micro-preemie in October of 2004.

My husband was taken on a tour of the NICU and shown babies at various stages of gestation. We were informed about Mitchell's chances of survival as well as the possible birth defects and mental disabilities he could face as the result of his premature birth. After considering his very low odds of survival were he to be born in a trauma situation as opposed to a controlled environment, we felt our best option was to have him delivered by C-section.

Looking back, we won't ever know whether we made the right decision. But we acted upon the advice of the doctors and the information that was available to us. Perhaps you have already faced such a choice yourself. Or perhaps you were never given a choice, and all the aspects of your baby's premature birth were entirely beyond your control. Either way, it is a very difficult situation in which most parents feel powerless.

Upon performing my C-section, the surgeon found a blood clot the size of his own fist. To this day, we don't know whether the blood clot caused the premature birth or the premature contractions caused the blood clot.

Mitchell Robert Cameron was born on October 10, 2004, at 8:46 p.m. He weighed 1 lb, 9oz. and he was 12.4 inches long. He was the most beautiful baby I've ever seen: so tiny and perfect. I was wheeled by him on my way to recovery. They didn't know whether he would make it through the night... but he did.

That was our son -- a true fighter, as we were to see over and over again. In the recovery area, my family came in and congratulated John and me on our new little boy. We were both still in shock and not sure what to expect.

I was taken to my room in the nursery area. It dawned on me then that I couldn't have my baby with me. My baby was clinging to life in the Neonatal Intensive Care Unit. Groggy from the pain meds, I slept through the night.

The next morning, I was awake at 5:00 a.m., calling my best friend on the East coast to tell her the news: my baby was here! I was elated.

Why was she so frightened? I could hear it in her voice. I felt that everything was going to be okay, because my baby was here. I was on a natural high for the next few hours -- until I went down to visit Mitchell.

As I was wheeled through the newborn area, I saw it in the nurses' faces: *There goes the mother of the 24-weeker... poor thing.* Those nurses knew something that I didn't -- which was how drastically my life would change over the next few months.

Kristy Cameron

2. How to survive your days inside the NICU

My hope is that you will learn from our experience so you'll have more time to enjoy your baby and need less time to learn the way of life in the NICU.

First Impressions

The first time you enter the NICU, you won't be on your feet. To this day, I remember rolling in the wheelchair up to the locked NICU door. I was still disoriented from Mitchell's birth and trying to hold on to any trace of sanity that might still be available to me. I was sitting at the door of my new life, waiting for a staff member to buzz me in. After my husband and I gave our names and were admitted, he rolled me down the long white hall to a huge washbasin where I would wash my hands hundreds of times. We had arrived in a completely foreign area of the hospital where each baby clings to life.

I was so focused on Mitchell that I didn't hear the beeping of monitors and alarms. I was the new kid on the block and I would learn fast that, as much as other NICU parents might want to know about your baby… no one will ask. Privacy is closely guarded here.

As I rolled across the room, time seemed to slow. I couldn't get to my baby quickly enough.

Finally we arrived at Mitchell's isolette and I longed to pick him up… but I couldn't because he was hooked up to a breathing tube, IV, feeding tube, heart monitor, blood pressure cuff, and an oxygen monitor. But underneath all of the life support equipment was the most beautiful baby I had ever seen.

If you are lucky, you might be able to touch your baby, but this is unlikely as micro-preemies are easily over-stimulated and have just been through an unexpected birth.

So there I sat, parked in my wheelchair, looking through the plastic wall of the isolette and longing to touch the miracle before me.

The doctors call the first two days of a micro-preemie's life *the honeymoon phase*. This is because the baby will not usually show many signs of distress, having been so recently supported by you. I think it's also called the honeymoon phase because, as parents, you have a brand-new premature baby and don't know what you're in for.

Two other phrases you will hear again and again are *roller-coaster* and *all right*. "Roller-coaster" refers to the inevitable ups and downs your baby will experience on a day-to-day basis. But as another parent of a preemie pointed out, riding a roller-coaster is fun and it happens by choice. The parents of preemies have been given no such choice and for me, the term became annoying and frustrating to hear.

I also learned that "all right" is the single most frequent phrase used to describe how your baby is doing. We eventually understood that the interpretation of these words depended upon the tone and inflection used by the hospital staff. If Mitchell was doing well, it was a quick, upbeat "all right." If he was having a rough day, it was often a drawn-out, heavier and cautious "all right."

The one piece of advice I can offer is not to take a minute for granted. Spend time with your baby. Talk to him and tell him over and over how much you love him. Your baby will know you are there.

At times I felt as if Mitchell wasn't my own baby because I had to get the nurses' permission to do anything for him. You may feel this way too, but just remember that it *is* your baby and the nurses are there to help both of you. They have seen and dealt with a lot, so take advantage of their experience and knowledge. They do truly care about you and your baby. I wouldn't have made it through this experience without the kindness, support, and compassion of Mitchell's nurses.

Friends & Family - Communication

Everyone in our group of friends and family wanted to know how Mitchell was doing on a daily basis. They were so supportive and worried about him that they wanted constant updates. As parents, we found ourselves overwhelmed by trying to communicate with everyone while also coping with Mitchell's situation.

Some of the best advice we received about communication was from an employee of the hospital. She gave us ideas on how to quickly spread information about Mitchell's condition while allowing us to remain focused on him. These two ideas may be the key to your sanity: a phone tree and e-mail. They sound simple enough, but in your fragile emotional state, simplicity can be elusive.

E-mail was our salvation. Once a week, I would send out e-mails detailing Mitchell's successes and challenges. The responses I received from people gave me strength. It was deeply comforting to know how many people were praying for him. It also made us realize how many people truly cared about Mitchell's progress.

I began adding people whom I didn't even know (friends of friends or family members) to the list and I'd receive e-mails from them offering prayers and encouragement. Use e-mail as a source of support. People are very kind and concerned and will share their thoughts and prayers for your little one.

We also found that by creating a phone tree (in which we ourselves only needed to call one person), we saved a lot of energy while still managing to keep everyone in our immediate families informed. By now you may have realized how desperately you need your energy. I think I went on auto-pilot at some point because I was so exhausted from worry and lack of sleep.

Another option that has emerged is the CarePages website. This patient-based website allows you to enter updates and photos without having to send emails. Your family may log in whenever they wish and automatically see the new postings and photos you have uploaded. It is very user-friendly, so even those of you who aren't completely comfortable with computers should be able to navigate the process without difficulty. It is a fantastic advancement in communication, and your support network will appreciate having constant access to the latest information about your baby.

Finally, you can also set up a private Facebook page and invite those you want to share your new baby with, including pictures and updates. At the time we had Mitchell this wasn't an option so you can see from the previous paragraphs it was a bit more complicated.

The point is to streamline your communication so you don't have to repeat the same information. Whatever method you decide to use, remember that you are only one person (or two with your spouse) and it will be terribly draining if you try to contact each member of your support network yourself.

You need to save your energy and strength for your baby.

Note

To make this book complete and give it a personal touch, I decided to include the e-mails that I sent out to our friends and family.

Not only do they reveal all the medical information and procedures relevant to Mitchell's journey, but hopefully they will also reinforce the idea that you are not alone in your experience with your new baby.

I hope it will give you some peace of mind to know that many other parents have been where you are right now and have survived the experience.

Regarding Mitchell – Update 1

Hi everyone...

I have decided to send out e-mails every few days to update you all on Mitchell's condition. I know for some of you it will be repeat information if John or I happen to talk to you but I think it will help me out in keeping everyone updated. Please feel free to call or visit anytime though because we love chatting and it does keep our spirits positive to feel the support that you have all offered.

As of Saturday evening Mitchell is doing well. He turned 25 weeks today and is going through "everything that is normal for a preemie" as the doctors say. His lungs are his biggest challenge and will continue to be for many weeks to come. When the nurses say it is a roller-coaster ride that we will be on for the next 3 months, they aren't kidding... there are lots of ups and downs.

On Friday, Charlie met his brother for the first time and actually got to touch Mitchell's leg. We took some pictures and I will send one out when they are developed. It was truly a great experience.

Mitchell is really cute and already developing a personality. The nurses say he is one feisty little guy who doesn't want to lie still for long periods of time. John has changed his diaper twice and we have been able to touch him a couple of times. He actually grabbed my thumb and held it for about 10 minutes the other day.

Thank you again for all the phone calls and support that you have offered. It means a lot to both John and I that we have so many friends and family that are there for us.

Love,
Kristy

Feelings of helplessness

We were the proud parents of a little baby boy and desperately wanted to protect him. Having our baby in the NICU left us with intense feelings of helplessness and it was easy to feel overwhelmed. My husband and I had to remember that, no matter what happened, we couldn't personally fix what was wrong.

If and when you become overwhelmed by these feelings, just know that you are not alone. Ask the nurses to put you in contact with other parents who have gone through the same experience, whether they are currently in the NICU or have been in the past.

I remember watching my husband sit and stare at Mitchell's monitors as if he were willing them to stay stable. He felt helpless to change the situation and needed to do something… anything. What we both ended up doing was looking at Mitchell's chart and learning as much as we could about his condition, prognosis, and any other information that could be relevant to his situation. This not only helped us to make more informed decisions about his care, but to some extent it helped alleviate the fear of the unknown.

We also spoke over the phone with the family of an 8-year-old boy who had been a micro-preemie. Talking with his father reminded us that we weren't alone in our experience, despite the fact that we often felt that way.

I say this again because it is so important: if you or your spouse feel lost or overwhelmed by your situation, ask a nurse to connect you with someone who has experienced the premature birth of a baby.   Or check to see whether there is a Family Advisory Group specifically designed to aid current NICU parents.   Even if you doubt you have the energy to do this, do it anyway... I promise that it will help. Even if your interaction with this person is limited to the phone, give yourself the gift of connecting with someone who has been where you are now.

How to Cope

There is nothing I can say that can truly alleviate the difficulty of what you're going through, except that I have been there and I know exactly how you feel.

Every person has a different response to stress. As I mentioned, we learned as much about preemies -- specifically in relation to Mitchell's health -- as we could to help us cope with our situation. I'm sure his doctors and nurses often felt as though they were conducting a medical seminar when they spoke to us, but we had a lot of questions. Every day we read Mitchell's chart so we would know as much as possible about his current condition and prognosis.

We also had the nurses take the time to teach us what the different tubes and machines did and how to interpret the monitors. It allowed us to understand what was happening with Mitchell without constantly having to ask someone else. The more you learn, the more you will understand about your baby's condition.

Another way to cope is to try writing in a journal. Even if you haven't written before, get a journal and write down your feelings. You can document the procedures your baby is undergoing and how you feel about everything that's happening.

I would write down things that I wanted to tell Mitchell when he was older, as well as the special things that happened during the times that I was with him. Not only will you preserve some cherished memories by doing this, but you might also find that it relieves some stress.

Writing in a journal can offer you a very private outlet for the joy, fear, doubt and many other emotions you might be feeling without repercussions from anyone. If you don't think you can take another minute of the madness, write it down. I guarantee you won't remember a lot of what is happening when it is all over. I was amazed by all our different experiences with Mitchell when I went back and read my journal entries. I am so glad now that I committed those experiences and emotions to paper.

Another way I coped was by reading to Mitchell. He liked Winnie the Pooh stories and we experienced all of Pooh's antics together. I'm sure he would have laughed if he could have. These stories and the experience of reading to my baby are memories that I will treasure forever.

If you ever sang while you were pregnant (or even if you didn't), try it now. While I was pregnant with Mitchell, I would sing "Rubber Ducky" to his older brother whenever he took a bath. Each day before leaving the NICU, I would sing "Rubber Ducky" to Mitchell and he would respond positively to the song and to my voice. Babies recognize their mothers' voices, so be sure to talk, read, or sing to yours on a consistent basis.

I wish with all my heart that I could give you an easy way to get through this experience, but I know that isn't possible. It is a tough road that you are traveling. Just remember to do your best and to take it all one day at a time. That is all anyone can ask.

Mitchell Update, 10/18

Hi, everyone!!!

Just wanted to send out an update on how Mitchell is doing and what has been going on the last few days. A little bit of background: all babies have a special blood vessel before they are born called a "PDA" that is responsible for transporting blood from the right side of the heart, bypassing the nonfunctioning lungs of the baby, and putting it directly into the aorta for circulation to the baby's tissues and organs. Before a baby is born, the mother's hormones close off the artery. In preemies, this artery isn't closed off and it fills the unformed lungs with a fluid that makes it difficult for the infant to get oxygen into his system (a tiny bit of medical info for you).

The last couple of days, Mitchell has been on medication to close off this artery. If the medication didn't work, he would have needed surgery to place a clamp on the artery. When we got to the hospital today, we learned that the medication worked and his artery closed!!! Yeah!!! That was great news.

The medication works by decreasing the size of his blood vessels, including the ones that go to his kidneys (sometimes the drug leads to kidney failure).

Consequently, he didn't have a wet diaper for two days... poor little thing. He was getting rather puffy from all the liquid that was building up in him and the nurses and doctors kept checking his tiny (and I mean tiny) diaper to see if anything happened. Tonight when we walked back in, his nurse was in the process of changing some things and on top of his incubator was a very wet diaper. I think it was the first time John and I have ever done a high-five over a wet diaper!

Things are going really well for him at this point and hopefully will continue to progress in that direction. Thank you everyone for your warm thoughts and prayers. I know they are helping him.

I've attached two photos: one with John's hand, so you can see how big Mitchell is and the other of just Mitchell. He has quite a few tubes and monitors attached to him, just to let you know before you look. The sunglasses are because he was under a photo lamp for several days to help a bit of jaundice that has since cleared up.

Kristy Cameron

Tonight when we were leaving, John and I were both staring in and said goodbye to him. He moved his fingers up and down twice like he was waving goodbye to us. I know it was a random thing but it brought tears to my eyes and smiles to our faces.

Lots of love to everyone...
Kristy

Awareness of what your baby is experiencing

As a parent, I'm sure you are aware that when you touch or talk to your baby, he or she can feel your love. For mothers, the connection has been there since before the baby was born. For fathers, it develops over time, and maybe it began the first time you laid proud eyes on your new baby.

In any case, showering your baby with love will help improve his condition. Of course, this alone won't cure all the ailments associated with premature birth. But as adults, we certainly feel better when we know our loved ones are there if we need them, so help your baby in this way too.

We weren't able to hold Mitchell at first, but he would grab my finger with his tiny fist. In this way, we were able to communicate through touch. It was important to me that he knew I was consistently there with him.

After a couple of weeks, when Mitchell became more stable, we did "kangaroo care" with him. For those of you who are unfamiliar with that term, imagine the following scenario:

You are reclining on your back with your shirt or blouse open and your skin exposed. You feel a little chilly while you are waiting for the nurses to lift your baby out of the isolette. (I was terrified that something would happen to Mitchell in the process, so I think I held my breath the whole time.) The nurses gently carry your baby over and lay him face to face with you. His warm skin touches yours for the first time. It's amazing.

I was so happy that tears were streaming down my face. The love and bonding you experience during that short span of time is absolutely magnificent and can't fully be described with words.

Studies indicate that this helps babies tremendously in their quest to heal and grow. I would say it also helps parents bond with their little one and communicate their love through touch.

Ask your baby's nurse about this. I highly recommend engaging in "kangaroo care" as often as is safe for your baby.

Mitchell update, 10/23

Hi everyone!

Mitchell is doing great!!! He will be two weeks old tomorrow and for the past three days, things have been very stable. Thank you to everyone for all the prayers and well wishes you have been sending. They are working!

Yesterday the doctor took out the tube that ran into his umbilical cord, so he is now being fed through an IV in his arm just like an adult. His heart rate and blood pressure seem pretty stable and his ventilator settings have been coming down (which is a very good thing). Mitchell has gained two ounces in the last 24 hours, which is another big step forward.

On Wednesday evening, the nurses changed the tube that goes into his mouth and they let me (for the first time) see what he looked like without any tubes or sunglasses on his face. He is a beautiful little guy and I just wanted to pick him up and give him a big love. He is also trying to open his eyes. It will be so awesome to walk in one day and find him looking back at us (even though all he will see are shadows for a while). For now, he recognizes our voices and actually responds when I sing "Rubber Ducky" to him. Charlie laughs when I sing it during his bath and I think Mitchell has heard it so often that it is already programmed into his brain.

That's all for now... please keep your prayers and good thoughts coming. John and I appreciate them more than you know.

Lots of love to everyone...
Kristy

Mitchell – a quick update

Hi everyone...

We just found out a few minutes ago that Mitchell pooped for the first time last night!!! His intestinal system is working!!! That will take more stress off his other systems and allow him to become stronger.

Just wanted to share the good news!

Love,
Kristy

Photos

From our experience, I have one word of advice for you: photos! Take lots of photos of your baby. Take photos of your baby with family members. Your baby's life has begun, so start celebrating it now! John and I took photos of Mitchell whenever his isolette was open and even through the open holes in the side.

One fun suggestion, offered by a nurse, is to place something (like a stuffed animal) beside your baby and take a photo every few days so you can see how much he is growing throughout his stay in the NICU. It will help reinforce your awareness of the progress your baby is making.

We also brought a picture of our family and hung it inside Mitchell's isolette. It gave him something to focus on and also helped staff members to recognize us when we were in the unit.

Mitchell update, 10/26

Hi everyone...

Here is some news on our little Mitchell. His doctor told us that preemies tend to have four major things that can and usually do happen to them... problems with the heart, lungs, brain, or intestines. She is amazed that Mitchell only has one problem which is his lungs. Actually the fact is that he doesn't really have any lungs yet since he was born so early. There are two sacs where his lung tissue is starting to grow. The ventilator, which keeps him breathing, also damages the lung tissue because it is so fragile... so it is a fine balance for the nurses to keep "the vent" at the ever-changing "correct" setting which will allow him to breathe without doing too much damage.

His lung condition isn't getting any better so they are starting five days of steroid treatment to try to get him off the vent. They say most babies respond well to this, with few side effects down the road. We are praying this will work so he will be on his way to a strong recovery.

A couple of positive things have happened. One is that Mitchell opened his eyes!!! His nurse saw it happen yesterday morning and has been poised with a camera (for two 12-hour shifts) waiting for her chance to snap a photo. The nurses in the NICU are wonderful. They treat Mitchell, John and I like family (that's just a side note for you).

Anyway, John and I saw him open his eyes today for the first time. It was sooo neat! He actually looked at us... yawned and stretched... and then closed his eyes and went back to sleep. Talk about huge grins on our faces!

Another positive thing that Mitchell has done is gain weight. He weighs 1lb 13.5 ounces and is closing in on the 2lb mark rather quickly. His fluid intake for the first several days was just an IV solution with all his nutrients, but they have gradually started feeding him milk. Now half his fluid intake is milk, which -- from what I have read in books -- is the best thing for him. Hopefully he will continue to put on weight and become a strong little guy.

I have attached a couple of photos. One shows the back of his head and how much black hair he already has. I think he is going to look like his dad. Yeah! The other two photos were taken when his eyes were open. (Again, there are lots of tubes and a skin abrasion where a tube was formerly attached in these photos.)

Wow... I didn't realize this e-mail was so long. I think it really helps me to send these updates out and tell everyone what he is up to. Thank you so much for caring so much about Mitchell. I am making him a journal of this whole experience and he will truly know how much love and concern was expressed from everyone. Thank you for all your prayers -- John and I really appreciate them.

Kristy

P.S. Thanks for all the funny responses to the "poop" e-mail!!!

Help From Others

You may feel as if your world has suddenly come to a screeching halt while everyone else is going on with their lives. This may make you feel alone, but please remember that you aren't. I can't say this often enough. **You are not alone!**

John and I found that our family and friends were willing to do whatever we needed to help us during this time. Often people want to help but aren't sure what you need. When friends and family ask what they can do, your natural response might be "Nothing," or "I can't think of anything right now." Stop right there! Everyone will benefit if you take this opportunity to give them something to do.

Even if you have to initiate the request for help, do it. Trust me, it took every ounce of energy to focus on Mitchell and to manage my emotions. Chores such as cleaning, laundry, and paying bills were the last thing on my mind. Even eating was a chore that took energy. Giving people the opportunity to show kindness will help them feel better while truly making your life easier... I promise.

Moreover, there are usually non-profit organizations affiliated with the hospital that offer support to families like ours. The nurses in the unit can give you these referrals.

If you don't have family around you for support, keep in mind that the nurses care tremendously and will support you as much as possible. Talking with them daily and getting to know them during the two months we were in the NICU helped me in so many ways. I know they truly cared about Mitchell and they were there for my husband and me when we needed a shoulder to cry on. They were also there to share the laughter when Mitchell did something cute.

The nurses have a lot of experience and knowledge. They are more than willing to answer questions and help you cope with your emotions. Most nurses have seen a lot and will help you in any way they can. Some of them may come to seem like family to you.

Ups & Downs

It is truly incredible to consider how many ups and downs we experienced. Mitchell's condition changed not only on a daily basis but sometimes by the hour and even by the minute.

One moment he would be in a very vulnerable state and the next, very stable. This may be hard to believe, but trust me, such fluctuations are common. The staff may have told you that your days will be filled with ups and downs, and very often, they are.

There were days when Mitchell would open his eyes and look at me or grab my thumb and hang on. I loved those moments and they would carry me through the bad times -- like the day that an infection set in and Mitchell was on six different antibiotics. The doctors had to remove his feeding tube and when they tried to give him an IV, his veins kept blowing. We almost lost him but he pulled through and overcame the infection. That was our little Mitchell: a true warrior.

On one of our happiest days, Mitchell went from the ventilator, which breathes for the baby, to CPAP which pushes air into the baby's lungs but allows them to breathe on their own. CPAP stands for Continuous Positive Airway Pressure and represents the next step on the road to recovery.

John and I stood there in the NICU and watched as they took Mitchell off the vent and put him on CPAP with absolutely no problems. He was breathing on his own! We were so proud of him that we literally jumped for joy! So although you will have your ups and downs, try to let go of the anguish of the darkest hours once they have passed, while focusing on – and celebrating – all that is positive and hopeful about your baby's situation.

Mitchell update, 11/1

Hello everyone...

It has been a while since I've sent an update but things have been very up and down over the last week. Mitchell is doing pretty well but there have been a couple of things that have happened to slow down his progress.

Hop on and I will let you experience the roller-coaster of Mitchell's progress. As I said in the previous e-mail, Mitchell started his five-day steroid therapy to mature his lungs enough to come off the ventilator. After three days of treatment, he wasn't responding and his doctor basically told us that we were going to have to "ride it out" and rely on the vent to get Mitchell through while hoping that it didn't do too much damage to his lungs. He gave Mitchell a 50/50 chance of survival. That was very devastating news since we were hoping the steroids would get him off the vent and on his way to a full recovery with healthy lungs.

At the same time his PDA (the heart artery) had re-opened a tiny bit, causing a heart murmur. If this had been worse, they would have had to do surgery to close it off... which would have been a huge setback. Thank goodness the murmur is now gone and things on that front are okay!!!
Two days ago his doctor told us that he has a hernia which will require surgery before he leaves the hospital. Believe it or not, they tell us this isn't

a huge concern... it is a simple operation and it won't be done until he is strong and able to take it. In the next breath, she told us some great news: Mitchell is, in her words, a very active baby who is aware of what is going on around him. This is unusual in 24-weekers (this is what they call him). Mitchell is soooo cute... he will open his eyes and lie there checking things out. I'm not sure he can actually see anything but shadows at this point but he is sure interested in what is going on around him. I can't imagine what he must be thinking right now, after going from a warm, safe, dark womb to an environment with all the machines beeping and lights shining on him.... probably "Put me back!!!"

Today there is more news and like all days... some of it is good and some of it is bad. The good news is they increased his last couple of doses of steroids and he is responding very well!!! When I walked in today, I actually had an adrenaline rush. He was breathing room air (which is 21% oxygen) with the help of the vent. They have brought down his vent settings and are optimistically hoping to get him off toward the end of the week!!!

The other news is he has a staph infection in his blood and possibly in his spinal fluid. He also hasn't had any stools (I guess that is the nicest way to say it) for the last four days, which puts him at risk for developing a disorder called necrotizing enterocolitis (NEC). This is an inflammation of the intestines caused by the fact that they are so immature and can't process the milk with the supplement they are adding. In worst-case scenarios, kids need surgery to correct this because the intestines rupture and leak into the body cavity. If Mitchell does have this... they have caught it early enough and started antibiotics so hopefully it will disappear within the next several days without any serious consequences.

Even though Mitchell is going through a lot right now, the fact that his lungs are improving so much is enough to keep us very positive about his prognosis. Mitchell held my finger today and I have to say he has quite the little grip on him for a tiny guy. He is a fighter and I know he will make it through this ordeal. Thank you for your prayers and positive e-mails that you have been sending. John and I appreciate all the cards, phone calls, offers of help, prayers and everything else that you all have done to support us. It truly does give us strength.

All our love,
Kristy

P.S. The photo is Mitchell at three weeks... the round Velcro on his head is for the sunglasses they attach when he has photo therapy... sometimes his little ear gets folded because his cartilage hasn't grown yet.

Hope

Never give up hope. Never. Whenever there is a bad day, there is almost always a good day to follow. Listen to the nurses when they tell you that your baby can sense your emotions. Always walk into the NICU with a positive attitude. Hope is everything. Don't let fear overpower you. It's not good for you and it's certainly not good for your baby.

That doesn't mean you won't feel fear and despair, because all parents do in a crisis involving their child. Just do your best not to let it dominate you. When it does threaten to overwhelm you, take a deep breath and try to focus on something positive. Believe me; I know this is much easier to read than to do.

But the more positive you can manage to stay, the better you will feel and the more positive energy you will offer to your baby.

Hope is powerful.

Mitchell update, 11/7

Hi everyone...

Well, it has been another of those weeks... up and down. John and I started the week thinking that Mitch would come off the ventilator by Monday or Tuesday at the latest. But as we all know by now, what we think and what really happens are two different things.

Mitchell responded very well to the second round of steroids. His vent settings were coming down several times a day and the docs were very optimistic about trying to wean him off the vent. John and I left the hospital on Monday with huge grins on our faces because we were certain that "the vent" would not be in our daily conversations after Tuesday. Can I just say... roller-coaster?

Tuesday morning we found out his staph infection was worse and the vent would be breathing for Mitchell for a few more days until the infection cleared. I believe it was Wednesday that they did a spinal tap and drew out some fluid to make sure he didn't have meningitis because his infection wasn't getting any better. Thursday rolled around and the infectious disease specialist came up and did an evaluation... by the end of Thursday, Mitchell was being injected with six different antibiotics. His blood cultures were still growing "colonies" of bacteria.

By this time getting off the vent was the least of our worries. It is funny how much more helpless you feel when you can't actually see if things are getting better or worse. At least with his lungs we can watch his progress, tell whether things are improving or not, and know what is going on. With his infections, we were completely in the dark and it was just a matter of waiting for the cultures to grow or not. By Friday morning, the third round of cultures came back positive for bacteria and so his main line (the tube which feeds him and administers his medicines) had to be pulled out. We have now learned that bacteria loves to grow on plastic and Mitchell's infection wouldn't clear up because it was in his tube too. Let me just tell you... Friday was the worst day we have had so far... by a long shot.

Before they could pull out his plastic tube, they had to start an IV so there would be a way to get all his meds and food into him. Close your eyes and imagine how small the veins of a 2-lb baby are... two different nurses tried and couldn't get an IV to stay. The nurses call it "blowing" when they try to put in an IV and the vein bursts. Mitchell had four veins blow with the two nurses. Finally, an off-duty nurse who happened to be in the unit for a meeting was able to get one vein to hold.

The next crucial thing we had to hope for was that this vein didn't blow for 24 hours. That was the length of time the docs wanted him free of plastic so the antibiotics could do their job. His next step was going to be surgery to insert a Broviac into his jugular vein. (A Broviac is a type of tube they use for long-term treatment that is sutured in under the skin.) The problem we were facing was that this is plastic and couldn't be placed until the 24-hour period was over. The first IV lasted for 3 hours and then blew. Another nurse found two more veins and they held overnight so we were into Saturday and ready for surgery!

I know it is a strange thing to be excited about surgery... but when you see your little baby lying there being pricked over and over, it tears at your heart. His little body is pretty bruised up from the ordeal. Surgery happened Saturday and the tube was inserted. Mitchell's surgeon said that pound for pound, he is a tough little guy and was very stable during the entire surgery. Right now he is doing great!!! They did blood cultures after surgery and 24 hours later, no bacteria have grown. This is such a positive thing!!!

His doc called this afternoon and said they are looking to start weaning him off the vent in the next 24-48 hours... so here we are again. We have come full circle and are hoping that by Monday or Tuesday, Mitchell will be weaned from the vent and it won't be in our daily vocabulary anymore.

It warms my heart when we walk up to his bed and his little eyes are staring back at us. His oxygen levels go up when either John or I touch him, which means he is happy!!!! He definitely knows

Mommy and Daddy and hopefully, very soon, we will be able to pick him up for the first time!!!

All our love to everyone,
Kristy

Mitchell -- another quick update

Hi everyone...

I held Mitchell for the first time tonight!!! They laid him on my chest with only his diaper on so he would feel my skin against his and then put a couple of blankets on top of him so he stayed warm. It was so incredible!!! I held him for a little over an hour. When they put him back in his incubator, the nurse said he looked more relaxed than she had ever seen him. I think it did both of us a lot of good.

I just wanted to share the good news...

Love,
Kristy

Just for Moms

High levels of stress keep your milk supply low. Here are some tips that the hospital's lactation specialists passed on to me. They will help if you are only pumping and can't nurse your baby yet.

- Eat avocados! One per day will increase your milk supply.

- Drink plenty of water. Carry a sports bottle with you at all times. If you get tired of water, mix it up with powdered tea or fruit flavoring.

- Pump every 2-3 hours around the clock, with the exception of one 5- hour stretch of sleep at night.

- Being around your baby stimulates your milk production. Always try to pump during a visit to the hospital.

- Eat as healthily as possible. Your baby eats what you eat.

- Keep taking your pre-natal vitamins (confirm this with your doctor).

- Even if you happen to catch a cold, keep pumping. You won't pass your cold to your baby through breast milk. In fact, your body will produce antibodies that will help protect your baby.

Every hospital has lactation specialists. Don't hesitate to approach them with any questions or concerns you may have. That's why they are there!

Mitchell update, 11/12

Hi, everyone...

Holy cow, what a week!!! This week has been very eventful... with most of the developments being positive which was nice and calming for all of us. Last Saturday, our pastor met us at the hospital and baptized Mitchell. It was a very moving experience.

On Sunday, Mitch spent most of the day recovering from surgery. Gosh, that seems like so long ago. His vitals were stable very soon after the surgery and several docs and nurses told us what a fighter he is. On Tuesday morning when I walked in, his doc was deciding whether or not to attempt to take him off the vent. As she talked, she decided we would give it a try. John left work and came down to the hospital.

Mitchell's doctor spent about ten minutes telling us it wasn't going to be a fun thing to watch. Preemies that haven't had to breathe on their own before will take a few breaths and then forget to breathe so the nurses usually have to resuscitate them. The picture I had in my head after this talk was of one of the nurses scrambling to get him to breathe and lots of frantic activity around his bed. The respiratory therapist came over and set up his CPAP (this is a machine that forces air up into his nasal passages... it keeps his lungs open slightly so it's easier to breathe). Everything was in place and John and I were holding our breath.

*They opened up his incubator and took the
ventilator tube out of his throat. John got to see
what he looked like without anything on his face
for the first time. It was fun to watch the proud
expression that crossed John's face while he was
looking at Mitchell. I think we may have taken a
picture of Mitch while he didn't have anything on
his face (along with several pictures of the floor in
all the excitement). I will attach it to the next e-
mail if it turns out.*

*Anyway, after they took the vent tube out of his
throat, they placed the CPAP tubes in his nose.
John and I waited for the flurry of activity to come.
I'm happy to say it never happened. Mitchell
started breathing on his own!!! The staff was as
excited as we were. Especially since they had two
nervous parents watching! His doctor built us up
for an excruciating experience and it was very
smooth and uneventful... which was fine with us.*

*Mitchell was doing wonderfully and John and I
were as happy as can be. We were finally on our
way to getting Mitchell on the road to recovery...
or so we thought. When there is a high, there is
always a low to follow. He did great on CPAP,
breathing on his own. The doctors were smiling
when they made rounds Wednesday morning.
Things were great when I left the hospital at 1:30
p.m. By 4:00 p.m. that same day, I was on the
phone with a surgeon because Mitch needed
emergency surgery. He had some serious swelling*

in his intestinal area and they weren't sure exactly what the problem was, so exploratory surgery had to be done. It turns out his intestines had a slight rupture and it caused some infectious material to collect in his scrotum.

It wasn't major surgery but they did have to put him back on the ventilator to do it. Once again... we are hoping to have him off the ventilator by Monday or Tuesday of next week. At least this time, we will know he has done okay on CPAP before and hopefully will do it again. The surgeon told us that at some point during the next three weeks or so, Mitchell will need surgery to correct the intestinal rupture... they think it closed off by itself but it will still need some repair.

Everything else is looking great. His little personality is shining through... tonight he made a mewling sound at the nurse because he was unhappy with her touching him to draw blood. A few of the nurses (there are 150 who work in the unit) are getting quite attached to him. One of his night nurses made a sign-up sheet for his care and attached it to his bed. It is filling up all the way through December! Oh... I almost forgot the most important thing... Mitchell was one month old on Wednesday!!!

Well, I'm off to bed now. Again, thank you for all the cards, e-mails, phone messages, and everything else you all are doing to support us. Each of you has touched us in your own way and helped us stay strong through this journey with Mitchell. Thank you...

Love,
Kristy

3. *Keeping up with life outside the NICU*

The Household

With everything that is happening inside the NICU, it is easy to forget that life does still go on outside of it.

You still have jobs to do, bills to pay, and possibly other children who need your attention. This all may be overwhelming and I wish I had an easy answer for you, but I don't.

The best advice I can offer is to take people up on their offers of help and be as organized as possible. If people don't know what they can do to help, here are some suggestions: laundry, general housecleaning, grocery shopping, providing care for your other children, and keeping people informed about your baby's condition.

Let people bring food over and freeze the dinners if need be. We were so grateful for these donated dinners as we started to wear down and had little energy for chores like grocery shopping or cooking. The longer your baby remains in the hospital, the more exhausted you may become, which is why your health is so important. I had so much worry and stress that I really had to focus on myself in order to stay as healthy as possible for Mitchell and the rest of my family.

Your Health

Eat and sleep. You may be thinking, "*Yeah, right.*" It is very hard to eat and sleep, but you have to try.

Make an effort to maintain a balanced diet so that when you are able to eat, your body is getting the nutrients it needs. If you are a mom and are pumping (which is highly recommended for preemies), drink lots of water and eat regularly. Missing meals can compromise your nutrition and affect your milk supply. Preemies need every advantage you can give them.

If you are a dad, help your wife to get adequate nutrition. She has just given birth and needs support. Taking care of her is one way you can help your baby. My own husband consistently expressed his frustration at not being able to help Mitchell. But in fact, he did help Mitchell by making sure I was eating and drinking properly so that my milk supply was sustained. It will be a challenge, but eat and sleep when you can... all you can do is your best.

Finally, I have said this over and over but it is so important: your emotions are probably raw and you might even find it hard to believe that all this is really happening. Let people help you in any way they can. Don't try to be heroic by doing everything yourself. You're in a frightening and unexpected place right now, so let others help you.

Anything that contributes to your own well-being can only benefit your baby.

Mitchell update, 11/20

Hi, everyone...

WOW!!! What a week this has been!!! We started off the week with a phone call from Mitchell's nurse telling us his oxygen needs were increasing even though he was on the vent. They moved him to a "high frequency" vent which pumps much faster and basically keeps his lungs open all the time instead of making them take breaths as ours do. To go to this vent is a step backward.

Mitchell stayed on the high frequency vent until Tuesday morning. He was still in a cycle where his body was demanding more help with oxygen... John and I were pretty freaked out by this time because Mitchell seemed to be heading in a very scary direction. His doc decided to move him back to his regular vent to try and get his respiratory system to respond. In the process (thank goodness we weren't there), his heart rate dropped drastically and they had to pull out his breathing tube and try to resuscitate him. When they pulled out his tube, they discovered it was blocked by some mucus from his lungs (as a side note... they have a procedure they do quite frequently that pulls out all of the mucus without any problems) so they were quite surprised by the blockage when they saw it. But not as surprised as they were by what happened next.
Mitchell started breathing on his own!!! So instead of placing him on his ventilator, they put him back on CPAP (continuous positive airway

pressure)... which, as you may remember, allows him to breathe on his own but also forces oxygen up his nose to help his little lungs out. I received a call from his doctor that I won't ever forget. I was standing in our kitchen when I answered and heard her voice. I almost fell over when she said Mitchell was back on CPAP. She started laughing and said (this is a direct quote), "Yep, Mitchell never ceases to surprise us." I couldn't help but laugh and jump up and down a couple of times!!!

He looked sooooo cute when we went to visit him. He was all tucked into his fleece blanket and had his Beanie Baby giraffe sitting right by him. But most importantly... he was still breathing on his own and it had been over six hours. They didn't know how long he could last because his lungs were sicker this time due to his surgeries, but as we all know by now... any time off the vent helps him produce important lung tissue.

That night was also special in another way: John held his son for the first time. It was very unexpected since Mitchell had just started breathing on his own again. The nurses had John take off his shirt and tip back in the recliner, then they laid Mitchell on his bare chest so they had skin-to-skin contact. The look on John's face was incredible and Mitchell's stats increased dramatically. They were both very happy... it was precious. John held him for about 45 minutes before he went back into his incubator.

On Thursday evening I got to hold Mitchell again!!! When I say hold, I actually mean I held him as if he were a big newborn baby!!! It was soooo incredible... it made me realize again how tiny he really is. But he looked so comfy lying there in my arms... I think he would have had a big smile on his face if he knew how to smile.

Well, since we all know the ups and downs of the NICU, we knew to expect a bit of not-so-good news. On Friday morning at 5:30 a.m., Mitchell's lungs began to tire out and he had to go back on the vent again. This isn't a bad thing because he just needed a break from working out his lungs.

We all are overjoyed that he lasted three whole days breathing on his own. His doctor said (you probably know what I'm going to say next) they think by next Monday or Tuesday he will be ready to come off the ventilator again.

I'm happy to say the rest of Mitchell (meaning everything other than his lungs) is doing really well... there are some concerns, of course, but things are looking good at this point. John and I pray that Mitchell will continue with his recovery and keep taking those big steps forward with only tiny ones back...

I know I say this with every e-mail I send out, but thank you to everyone for all the support that you are sending to our family... and especially to Mitchell. I wish every one of you could feel the strength and love that is being sent our way right now. It is truly amazing!!!

Love,
Kristy

Timing

Try to visit the hospital while the doctor is making rounds. Make sure to ask any questions that you might have. If you are inquisitive and really talk with the doctors daily, you will become familiar with, and understand, the medical terminology. I always felt it was important to understand what was happening so that we could make informed decisions regarding Mitchell's health.

Something else that we learned as our time in the NICU crept along is that the evenings were much quieter and more peaceful than the daytime hours. This may just have been my own personal preference, but I loved sitting with Mitchell during the evenings. I talked to him and cooed to him and felt that, without the daytime noise competing with my voice, he was able to listen more closely and enjoy our time together more.

Mitchell update, 11/28

Hi, everyone!

I hope you all had a great Thanksgiving and enjoyed the time spent with loved ones. This week has been so incredibly positive with Mitchell that I don't quite know where to start.

Mitchell has been growing like a weed! You won't believe this but he weighs 2lbs 10 oz now. I couldn't visit him for six days because I had a cold (it was so hard not to see or touch him for that long). I called and talked to the nurses a lot and John was very good at describing what Mitchell was up to. When I went back on Thanksgiving morning, I couldn't believe how much he had grown. His feet are huge and pack a powerful kick for a little guy (I found this out as I changed his diaper). His body is starting to create baby fat and he doesn't look quite so fragile anymore.

Mitch has also been on CPAP breathing on his own for the last five days!!! So far there haven't been any signs that he is tiring out. The most amazing thing about that is, we made it through a Friday and Saturday without Mitchell having to go back on the vent again!!! Yeah!!!

Last Tuesday Mitchell had his first eye exam and everything looks really good. He will continue to have exams every two weeks to check for ROP (which stands for retinopathy of prematurity, a potentially blinding disease affecting the retinas in premature infants). In infants born prematurely, the blood vessels that supply the retinas haven't fully developed and can grow into each other. So far Mitchell doesn't have any signs of this disease.

Finally, the most exciting news of all... Mitchell pooped. I know you may be thinking, "Yikes! That's exciting???" Yes... the doctor just called and told me, and you would have thought I had just won the lottery. John just walked in the house from Christmas shopping and when I told him, he started laughing and was literally dancing around!!!

What this means is that Mitchell's system is working and hopefully he won't need surgery to take out part of his intestines. This surgery is something that has been looming over our heads for the last four weeks. They kept saying he had a blockage, most likely from scar tissue that would need to be removed before his system would start working again.

Mitch is scheduled for an upper GI tomorrow morning and we will know more about any blockage then... but for now John and I are hoping that dirty diaper = no surgery. *I think that is all for now.*

Have a great week!!!

Love,
Kristy

The waiting game

Sitting and waiting… waiting and sitting. I stare into the isolette at my little angel fighting for his life. In the background, I can hear the seconds ticking by on the clock. My whole body is still but active at the same time. My mind reels from the agony of waiting for my baby to get well. My heart aches over the painful procedures he has to go through on an hourly basis. My body craves his touch, even for a brief minute. I want to reach in and touch him, skin to skin, but I am afraid I'll transfer germs to him or cause him more stimulation and duress than he can handle. So I sit beside his bed and pray that his strong will is enough to carry him through to recovery. I look at my beautiful baby underneath all the tape and tubes… still waiting… for time to pass and my baby to heal and grow.

You'll do this, too.

4. *Other NICU Stories*

~*contributed by Moms of Preemies*~

Jalesa Faith
as told by Mom LaCosta Herrion

I didn't plan on having any more children, so it came as a shock when I found out that I was nine weeks pregnant with Jalesa. I had a 10-year-old daughter and an 8-year-old son and I asked myself, *how in the world am I going to do this again?*

This pregnancy was different; I was always anxious. We had several ultrasounds but could never figure out the sex. After one particular appointment, I received a call from my OB/GYN that I was being referred to a specialist because my alpha-fetoprotein (AFP) test was abnormal. I had a 1 in 135 chance in having a baby with Down's syndrome. I wasn't that worried about it because this same scenario happened with my first child, a girl.

My husband and I went to see the same specialist that I saw ten years prior. We saw the doctor and he gave us the option of having an amniocentesis (amniotic fluid test) to determine whether or not she would have Down's syndrome. I was completely against it, but my husband insisted that I have the test done. I was so scared, but not for the results; I wanted my baby, regardless.

The test results came back fine and everything was going smoothly until my OB/GYN discovered that I was suffering from the early onset of hypertension. I started taking the blood pressure medications that I was prescribed and they worked for a few weeks.

However, by the time I hit 21 weeks, I felt terrible all of the time. It was so bad that I would frequently drive to the doctor's office and ask to be seen. It was fortunate that he was the one that delivered my other two children, so he knew what was abnormal for me.

At 23 weeks, my blood pressure was 220/120. He instantly called the hospital and admitted me. He stayed with me an entire week to check my progress. After the week was up, he decided to let me go home for the weekend and see how my swelling was the following Monday; I had two days to pray that everything went back to normal, which I hoped was the case, as I had older kids who needed me too.

Monday morning I went back to the hospital with higher blood pressure. My OB/GYN doctor (Dr. Deiter) asked if I had been getting steroid shots yet. I was so confused. *Steroid shots for what?* I had been doing everything that I was supposed to do. *Was I going to die, was the baby going to make it?*

I was going to be transferred to OU Children's Hospital where they were more equipped to handle premature births.

At this point I was 24 weeks into my pregnancy. The paramedic who was in charge of getting my vitals on the ride over to OU Children's Hospital was very pleasant. He shared with me that his granddaughter was born at 27 weeks and she was doing fine.

We said a little prayer while I was back there and I cried the rest of the way. Once we made it to the hospital, it was a battle to get my blood pressure down. I was told that it was possible that I had to have her that night. I simply replied, "No, she's not ready and neither am I!" I hadn't even picked out her middle name.

At that moment I heard a voice say, "Give her the middle name of Faith because you will need your faith to get you through this," and so I did. Thankfully, my hospital staff was able to keep her safely inside my belly for the time being. I had a wave of emotions, including neglect of my older children.

An ultrasound that indicated that the baby wasn't getting enough oxygen and that she was lacking blood flow to her placenta. The decision was up to me: deliver her now or continue to wait. I decided I wanted to continue on for as long as I could. My ex mother-in-law's birthday was coming up and I joked that we couldn't do it then. They all laughed.

That night, I learned that my liver was failing… one more reason to have her. I heard the little voice again. It said, "It's time for her to come out, trust me, she will be fine."

I had left the room and came back to six doctors, two neonatologists and eight nurses. If I continued the pregnancy, I was looking at a stillborn baby due to the fact that several portions of my placenta were unhealthy. My baby was definitely not getting any blood flow or oxygen to multiple areas and I hadn't eaten or had anything to drink in more than 12 hours.

Jalesa Faith was born at 11:15 a.m. on February 18, 2010. I had just started my 27th week of pregnancy. I didn't expect a cry because the neonatologists explained that she might not, but she cried! She sounded like a baby kitten meowing. I was so overjoyed.

My precious miracle weighed one pound eight ounces and was 13.5 inches long. She had hair! Jalesa Faith was so adorable. They let me look at her and then whisked her away to the NICU. Now it was time to get my health back. I spent the next week or so on bed rest in the hospital.

When it was time for me to leave, I cried and cried. I didn't want to leave my baby. Two weeks later, I finally got to hold her, but then she stopped breathing. I was terrified. I was always told to expect one step forward and two steps back while in the NICU and they were right about that.

Jalesa started out doing so well that she didn't have to be intubated, instead, she was on a CPAP machine. One day, around the time that she was two weeks old, I went in and heard a call about a baby coding. It was Jalesa. The nurse said, "This isn't like her, she's been doing this all day."

Her neonatologist pulled me aside and explained that she behaved as if she had an infection somewhere, but they couldn't find it. My baby was really sick. Her doctor said, "I have to be honest about this, we don't think she will make it."
Those words were so hard to hear, but I felt in my gut that she would be fine. I stated, "No, Jalesa will be fine. She is my baby and I have already been assured that she will grow up to be a healthy little girl."

I went on to explain to the medical staff that she had to have my attitude because my older daughter did. We later found out that she had pseudomonas, caused by common bacteria, and her lungs were getting less air because of it. They were "cautiously optimistic" that the antibiotics they put her on would clear it up, but it was a waiting game.

After about 10 days, she got better! No more high-pressure jet (a ventilator that delivers fresh air into the baby's lungs quickly) and mommy could finally hold her again! I was so excited to see her on regular oxygen. Time progressed and, finally, it was time for us to go home, but not without medical equipment.

After taking classes to find out more, I agreed to bring Jalesa home on a pulse oximeter monitor and an apnea monitor. "Miss Priss" came home on her due date of May 24, 2010, after 94 days of being in the NICU. It was such a happy day!

Jalesa has gone through physical, speech and now occupational therapy to get her to where she needs to be. She has a few health problems, such as chronic lung disease, but she is here!

She is still tiny. At four years old she weighs in at 31 pounds and 41 inches tall. She is in Pre-K now and I'm so proud of her. She amazes me every day! I wouldn't change this experience because it continues to make me a better person as the days go by.

Jalesa Faith is here for a reason. She's my miracle and the tiniest thing I ever put my whole heart into.

Kai & Matteo
as told by Mom Jimena Guild

My story begins early on in my pregnancy. At 14 weeks gestation, I was diagnosed with a Partial Placenta Previa. For those who don't know, it's when a portion of your cervix is covered by the placenta. Baby A had implanted on my cervix, so whenever his umbilical cord would pull on my cervix, I would bleed. Sometimes small bleeds, other times, full-on hemorrhages where I almost passed out from loss of blood.

The doctors kept telling me Previas usually fix themselves. As the placenta grows, it pulls away from the cervix, and your issues are resolved. Of course, that wasn't the case for me, as I had two babies, and baby B was lying across my stomach. He took up any room that baby A had to move up at all, so my Partial Previa eventually turned into complete Previa. There was no chance it would ever improve, and C-section was unavoidable.

I hemorrhaged seven times in 14 weeks – four of those times, it was enough for me to almost blackout. In the end, I had three blood transfusions.

At 26 weeks gestation, the doctors gave me the preventative steroid shots and prepared us for the strong possibility of these babies coming early. The last hemorrhage happened while I was on strict bed rest in the hospital, so the doctors decided for my safety; it was time to take the babies out. I had just hit 28 weeks gestation.

The statistics were really scary; nothing they were telling us was positive. Things like the babies may not make it, the very likely possibility of brain damage, brain bleeds, infections, cerebral palsy, etc. I remember halfway tuning them out because the sound of my heart beating was so loud, and my inner voice kept saying, "Why me? Why me? Wasn't my complicated pregnancy enough? Now to deal with having my babies come early?" As soon as they left, I broke down. This isn't how one envisions their pregnancy journey to be; filled with fear, frustration, worry, and sadness.

I think it had finally hit me, all the emotions I had bottled up from the entire journey so far. I had been strong through the whole thing, but being stuck in bed for almost 14 weeks, constant hospital emergency visits, six hemorrhages, and an early birth scare, there is only so much a person can carry on their shoulders, and I think I had finally reached my max.

People talk about postpartum depression; I think I had prepartum depression. I had hit an ultimate low. I couldn't even hear about other uneventful pregnancies, let alone watch a happy pregnant lady walk down the street without feeling total jealousy and anger. I had been robbed of everything I had always envisioned.

Barely anyone saw me pregnant since I was stuck in bed for most of it. I didn't get to flaunt my pregnancy as I dreamed, I never got to shop for pregnancy clothes, and never had pregnancy photos done like I wanted. What about my baby shower? It was devastating.

On August 14, 2011, via C-section, Kai was born weighing 971 grams. One minute later, Matteo came into the world weighing 2.1 lbs, both measuring 12.5" in length. They struggled to breathe on their own and needed the help of a ventilator. Sadly, as is the case for most, if not all, micro preemie births, I was not able to see them right away, as they had to be rushed into an incubator. My husband was able to see them while I stayed behind to rest.

I had mixed emotions knowing that two little babies had come out of me, and neither had been able to take advantage of the kangaroo care I had always envisioned (holding the naked or partially dressed child against the bare skin of a parent). It wasn't until 24 hours later that I was able to visit them in the NICU.

After all the research I had done online about premature birth, I thought I would be prepared for it all. I wasn't. Nothing can prepare a parent for the NICU roller coaster.

I couldn't help but burst into tears at the sight of them. I had started lactating so you can imagine the combination of those emotions with the first glimpse of your babies. I was seeing my babies through a glass enclosure and not able to hold them against my chest.

I could reach in one hand and rest it on their back, but no rubbing or caressing was allowed because they said it was too much stimuli for a preemie. Their skin is so thin and sensitive to touch; it would do more damage than good.

There were so many machines attached to them, IVs and central Peripherally inserted central catheter (PICC) lines going everywhere (a thin, soft, long catheter (tube) that is inserted into a vein in your child's arm, leg or neck. The tip of the catheter is positioned in a large vein that carries blood into the heart. The PICC line is used for long-term intravenous (IV) antibiotics, nutrition, or medications, and for blood draws), it was heartbreaking to see them this way.

While I was still in the hospital recovering, I would get nightly visits from the NICU residents asking for permission to do tests on our babies. From inserting a PICC line to having to do multiple brain scans to even a couple of spinal taps when there was a scare of meningitis looming over them.

I entered motherhood, drenched in fear and sadness. I didn't even want anyone besides our immediate family visiting me in the hospital during those first three days. I couldn't stand to have friends visit me and congratulate me with flowers. Congratulate me on bringing my fragile babies into the world so early? It was not a time to rejoice in our eyes. I'm glad I had a private room because having to share a place with a joyous couple holding their newborn baby would break me.

There aren't enough words to describe how gut-wrenching it is to give birth and then be discharged from the hospital empty-handed. For the first time in 28 weeks, I was going to be many kilometers away from them. I wouldn't be able to get out of bed and wander into the NICU at any hour of the day. It would require a lot more planning for that from now on. Our four-month NICU journey was only beginning we were to discover.

Both needed to be on a ventilator for the first few hours to stabilize them. Kai (baby A) was the smaller of the two and suffered more of the punches during those four months.

They were both born with a Patent ductus arteriosus (PDA) – a congenital heart defect common in premature babies in which the vessel connecting the pulmonary artery to the descending aorta fails to close. When this happens, it allows some of the baby's blood to bypass the lungs. If left untreated, a PDA can lead to pulmonary hypertension, cardiac arrhythmia (irregular heartbeat), and congestive heart failure. Matteo's PDA closed with the help of medication, but Kai required closed heart surgery when he was a month old to correct it.

Both kids were also born with Respiratory distress syndrome (RDS) and needed medication to help tackle it. As well, Matteo had severe problems with apnea. Many times while we were visiting them in the NICU, he would stop breathing, and the machines would start going off, and the nurses would come over and rub him and coach him to start breathing again. This happened a lot, he would go a good 20 seconds or more without responding, and each time you would think it would get easier for me to witness, but it never did.

They both had Intraventricular hemorrhage (IVH – bleeding in the brain), Matteo had a level one bleed and Kai had a level 2, so they required many brain scans to keep an eye on them make sure it wouldn't get worse.

It was a vicious circle. On top of it, both had to have their eyes checked regularly for Retinopathy of Prematurity (ROP) – abnormal growth of blood vessels in the eyes, which can lead to vision loss – common again for preemies before 32 weeks. The tests were terrifying to watch; the babies' screamed so much I couldn't be in the same room it was terrible. Luckily both kids had it mild with just a grade 1-2, and all that was needed was to be followed closely for the first year of life with a specialist.

Kai had bad anemia and needed two blood transfusions as well. Kai also developed an awful double inguinal hernia in his groin. Matteo ended up contracting pneumonia while in the NICU and was intubated for a week.

The twins struggled with feeds a lot. We tried multiple times with Matteo to get him off his nasal gastric (NG) tube, and finally, close to discharge; he started taking feeds orally. Sadly, because Kai was on continuous positive airway pressure (CPAP) for many weeks, we couldn't try oral feeds with him until he was stable. Even when he was stable, he struggled with the feeds and would refuse them orally. At one point after Matteo was discharged and Kai reached the "corrected age" of a newborn, the NICU allowed us to take Kai home with his NG tube after properly being trained on how to administer feeds and change his NG tube monthly. Bringing them home close to Christmas was amazing.

Matteo spent three and a half months in the NICU while Kai spent four. Visiting them felt surreal. We didn't feel like they were ours. I didn't feel like a mom. It wasn't until the twins came home that we finally were able to feel like parents. We knew the road for us was still not over; they were still preemies, and we'd have to keep them quarantined for a little while longer, especially in the middle of flu and RSV season.

My husband had accepted a new job shortly before I gave birth and so he was unable to take time off to help me at home. I struggled basically on my own (my in-laws lived over 12 hours away, and my parents were still working full time), not only having to learn the ropes with two preemies, but one being on a strict four-hour feeding schedule via his NG feeding machine. I won't lie; there were many days I would break down as soon as my husband would get home. I was mentally drained on a daily basis. Luckily, after a month of being at home, the hospital provided in-home nursing services for 12 months, two times a week, to assist with Kai's feeds.

Kai did not improve with his oral feeds, and we were referred to an occupational therapist (OT) who specialized in feeding issues with preemies. He would not take to the bottle or my breast and was diagnosed as having a severe oral aversion. Everything had to be through his NG tube. We had OT services once a week for 12 months.

Once I went back to work, we lost the nursing and OT services and relied on our learned skills and our daycare provider to assist us. Slowly Kai began to improve, and one day while at daycare, Matteo accidentally pulled Kai's NG tube out, and we decided to not put it back in as an attempt to see how well he did. With the help of his dietician (who also came weekly to weigh him and assess his diet), we slowly began to see improvements.

After two years on an NG tube, Kai finally kicked it for good! We were so happy! Changing the NG tube was awful; I always had to hold him down while my husband would fish the tube from his nose into his stomach. He hated the experience, and I couldn't blame him for it. Kai is an entirely different child now. Luckily he has no recollection of his NG experience and is an amazing eater – better than his brother!

We have HAPPILY been discharged from:
+ cardiology,
+ speech therapy (delayed speech brought on by their prematurity),
+ nephrology (Kai's constant calcium build up in his kidneys, also   brought on by prematurity),
+ NICU follow up appointments,
+ OT services,
+ Physiotherapy,
+ blood pressure medication,
+ NG tubes,
+ reflux medication,
+ PediaSure to increase weight,
+ nursing services, and finally,
+ the dietician.

The only ongoing issue we are dealing with is Kai has gastro problems. He isn't fully potty trained as he has dulled sensation (urge) to go to the washroom, so we visit monthly a gastroenterologist and have him on daily stool softeners with monthly enemas. Luckily this is something that will eventually resolve itself; we don't know when that will be.

We've come a long way, and looking back, I couldn't imagine making it this far today. The future looked so grim, and we felt so alone.

I want to let other parents know that you're definitely NOT alone and also to let you know that we've been there! Even though they may not be considered preemies by the standard medical book anymore, they will always be preemie warriors to us.

5. *Leaving the Hospital*

Walking out of the hospital with your baby in your arms is one of the most wonderful and frightening feelings in the world. You are now the person responsible for the health and care of your baby.

By the time you leave the hospital, you will know a lot about monitoring your baby as well as the meaning of many medical terms (such as O2 danger zones and Bradys) just from all the time you have spent at your baby's side.

But before you are allowed to take your baby home, you will attend some classes that will teach you how to monitor any machines or devices that your baby will need at home. These classes are very informative and the nurses will make sure you know exactly how to handle any situation that might arise. The nurses won't be at your home to help you if something happens, so make sure you have asked any questions you might have, and that you know what to do in an emergency. Many hospitals also require parents of premature babies to complete a course on first aid for infants.

Try to have a support system in place before you take your child home. This will alleviate some of the stress that will inevitably accompany this transfer of responsibility. Think of the emotional and physical strain you have been through and put that support in place even if you don't feel you will need any immediate help.

In spite of the apprehension you may be feeling, remember that this is the day you have dreamed of for weeks, possibly even for months. Celebrate and enjoy it! The newest member of your family is coming home.

A final note~

During Mitchell's stay in the hospital, his experiences offered lessons about life even to people who knew him only through e-mail or word of mouth. One of the most life-affirming messages I received during this ordeal was how helpful and generous others can be during a time of crisis.

Now, thanks to Mitchell and my experiences with him, I am able to help others in their time of need.

What is Mitchell's gift?
Mitchell's presence here led me to write this book for *you.*

6. *NICU Glossary*

The following glossary is a list of general definitions that I have found to be used in the NICU. They are meant to be used only as a means to understand and help you communicate within the unit.

To understand a diagnosis or episode that your baby may experience, I strongly urge you to consult with your neonatologist or NICU nurse.

A

ABO incompatibility
A possible blood incompatibility between the mother and the fetus.

Abduction
Abduction is the movement of an arm or leg away from the midline of the body. Abduction of both legs spreads the legs. The opposite of abduction is adduction; adduction of the legs brings them together.

Acidosis
The PH of the blood is abnormally low.

Adjusted Age
Another name is *corrected age.* This is your child's chronological age minus the number of weeks he or she was born early. For example, if your 10-month-old was born 2 months early, you can expect him or her to look and act like an 8-month old. Usually you can stop age-adjusting by the age of 2 or 3.

AGA (appropriate for gestational age)
The baby's birth weight was within the normal range for the time the baby was in the womb.

Alpha Feto Protein (AFP) - a protein which is produced by the fetus and can be measured prenatally in the mother's blood to identify possible birth defects.

Alternative birth center (ABC)
A hospital room with a warm homelike feel to it where a woman can experience a natural childbirth, recovery and postpartum stay.

Alveoli
The alveoli are tiny air sacs within the lungs where the exchange of oxygen and carbon dioxide takes place.

Amblyopia
A loss of vision, centered in the brain, that develops when the brain fails to receive proper signals from a weak eye.

Amniocentesis
A procedure to obtain a sample of amniotic fluid from the womb.

Amnioreduction
The removal of large volumes of amniotic fluid by amniocentesis.

Aminophylline
A medication used to stimulate an infants breathing. It is prescribed to reduce the incidence of apneic episodes.

Amniotic fluid
The fluid surrounding the fetus in the uterus, which protects the fetus during pregnancy.

Amnionitis
An infection of the amniotic fluid.

Ampicillin
An antibiotic used to treat a bacteria infection.

Anemia
Fewer red blood cells than normal levels in the baby. This makes it harder for the baby's bloodstream to deliver oxygen throughout the body.

Anomaly
A malformation of a part of the body.

Anoxia
A near absence of oxygen in the blood and body tissue.

Antibiotics
Medicines used to treat infection.

Antibodies
Proteins produced by the body that fight infections. Many helpful antibodies are found in a mother's breast milk, and can be passed into a baby through breast milk feedings.

Aorta
The largest artery in the body.

Apgar Score
A score of 0 to 10 given to baby at the time of birth to access how well it has transitioned to life outside the womb. Points are assigned beginning at one minute after birth, and at five-minute intervals thereafter, for heart rate, respiration, reflexes, muscle tone, and color, until an infant is stable.

Apnea
Cessation of breathing lasting 20 seconds or longer. Also known as an apneic episodes or apneic spells. It is common for premature infants to stop breathing for a few seconds. They almost always restart on their own, but occasionally they need stimulation or drug therapy to maintain regular breathing.

Appropriate for Gestational Age (AGA)
A baby whose birth weight falls within the normal range for his or her gestational age.

Areola
The dark area on the breast surrounding the nipple.

Arterial Blood Gases (ABG)
A sampling of blood obtained from an artery in order to analyze its oxygen, carbon dioxide, and acid content.

Arterial catheter (indwelling arterial catheter)
A thin plastic tube placed in an artery to give nutrients, and medications, measure blood pressure, and to withdraw blood for testing. Arterial catheters are most commonly placed in the umbilical artery.

Arteries
Any blood vessel that leads away from the heart. Arteries carry oxygen to all parts of the body.

Asphyxia
A lack of oxygen

Aspiration
1. breathing a foreign substance such as meconium, formula, or stomach contents into the lungs; may cause aspiration pneumonia. 2. withdrawal of material from the body by suctioning.

Asymmetric (head-sparing) growth restriction
When a small-for-gestational age, baby is born with a normal head circumference. Asymmetric growth restriction is believed to occur when nutrients are in short supply in the womb and nature preferentially gives scarce nourishment to the brain - a vital organ - compared to the rest of the body.

Atelectasis
Failure of full expansion of the lung at birth or a collapse thereafter of the lung.

Attending physician
A fully-trained physician in a teaching hospital in charge of some or all of the patients in the NICU.

Audiologist
A trained professional who tests for hearing loss in infants, assists in determining the cause of such hearing loss, and plans a program to address hearing impairment.

Audiometric testing
Tests for hearing loss.

B
Bagging
A mask is placed over the baby's mouth, and an attached plastic bag is squeezed to pump breaths of air into the baby's lungs.

Betamethasone
A steroid medication given to a mother when a premature delivery is anticipated to help the baby's lungs mature. It also helps intestines, kidneys, and other systems to mature.

Betamimetics (also called beta-adrenergic drugs or betasympathomimetic drugs)
A category of drugs used to stop labor.

Bacteria
One-celled organisms that can cause infection.

Bacterial vaginosis (BV)
An infection caused by the overgrowth of common bacteria which normally live in the vagina, it is believed to be a risk factor for preterm delivery.

BAER (Brainstem Auditory Evoked Response)
A painless test done to check an infant's hearing. Usually done by an audiologist just before or after discharge from the NICU.

Bicarbonate (bicarb), (sodium bicarbonate), (NaHCO3)
A substance given to a baby orally or intravenously to help neutralize excess acid in the blood.

b.i.d.
Seen on a prescription meaning "twice a day".

Bililights (phototherapy)
Special blue florescent lights used to treat neonatal jaundice.

Bilirubin
Yellow waste product formed when red blood cells breakdown. When bilirubin accumulates, it makes the skin and eyes look yellow, a condition called jaundice.

Bladder tap
Is a procedure to withdraw urine from the bladder under sterile conditions by inserting a needle through the abdominal wall directly into the bladder.

Blood Culture
A blood test to look for infection in the bloodstream of the baby.

Blood Gases
A blood test used to evaluate an infant's level of oxygen, and carbon dioxide in the blood. This test is significant because it helps to evaluate an infant's respiratory status.

Blood Glucose
A test used to determine the baby's blood sugar.

Blood group or type
The classification of blood based on the presence or absence of certain proteins. Each person belongs either to type O, A, B, or AB. Differences in blood type between mother and baby (ABO incompatibilities) can lead to anemia and jaundice in the baby.

Blood is also categorized as Rh positive or Rh negative by the presence or absence of the Rh factor. When an Rh negative mother carries an Rh positive child, antibodies in her blood may cross the placenta and attack her baby's red blood cells. The resulting condition, called erythroblastosis fetalis, is characterized by severe anemia and jaundice in the newborn.

Blood pressure
The force exerted by the circulating blood against the walls
of the blood vessels. It is this pressure that causes the blood
to flow through the arteries and veins. The blood pressure
measurement is given in the form of two numbers. The top
number, the systolic pressure, is the measurement of the
pressure exerted when the heart contracts and sends blood
to the body. The lower number, the diastolic pressure, is the
measurement of the pressure exerted during the relaxation
between heartbeats.

Blood Urea Nitrogen (BUN)
A blood test that measures how well the kidneys are
functioning.

Bonding
The process by which parents and baby become
emotionally attached.

BPD (bronchopulmonary dysplasia)
Lung disease or damage as a result of prematurity/
ventilator therapy.

Bradycardia ("Brady")
A slow heart rate. Medications (theophylline or caffeine)
are often used to treat these spells in newborn babies.

Brainstem Auditory Evoked Response Test
A hearing test where a tiny earphone is placed in the baby's
ear to deliver sound. Small sensors, taped to the baby's
head, send information to a machine that measures the
electrical activity in her brain in response to the sound.

Brain bleed
Bleeding or hemorrhaging into some part of the brain.

Brain death
An absence of electrical impulses from the brain.

Braxton-Hicks contractions
"Practice" contractions of the uterus. The contractions occur at irregular intervals during pregnancy and do not lead to effacement or dilation of the cervix.

Brazelton Neonatal Assessment Scale (BNAS)
Helps professionals assess the baby's pattern of response to their environment.

Breast milk fortifier
A Protein, vitamin, and mineral mixture which are mixed with breast milk

Breast milk jaundice
A common type of jaundice thought to be caused by a substance in the mother's milk.

Breech delivery
When a baby is born buttocks or feet first.

Brethine
Is used to quiet uterine contractions and slow or prevent premature delivery.

Bronchial tubes
The tubes that lead from the trachea (windpipe) to the lungs.

Bronchioles
Small tubes that branch off from the bronchial tubes.

Bronchiolitis
An inflammation or infection of the bronchioles.

Bronchitis
An inflammation or infection of the bronchial tubes.

Bronchoscopy
The use of an endoscope to examine and take biopsies from the interior of the bronchia

Bronchopulmonary Dysplasia (BPD)
Is lung damage and scarring that occurs in some babies who were treated with oxygen and the vent for a long period of time.

Broviac Catheter
Type of intravenous tube (central line) used to give fluids and medications to infants or children. The catheter is placed in a major vein of the body during surgery.

BUN (blood urea and nitrogen)
A blood test for liver and kidney function.

C
Caffeine
Used to treat apnea.
Caffeine citrate (Cafcit®)
A central nervous system stimulant that's used to treat certain breathing problems in premature infants. This medication is given intravenously.

Calcium
A chemical necessary for the normal functioning of the nerves, the heart, and other muscles, and for the growth of bones and teeth.

Candida albicans (monilia)
The fungus that causes thrush and other "yeast" infections.

Capillaries
Tiny blood vessels that come into close contact with the body cells to supply the cells with oxygen and nutrients, and to remove waster products.

Carbon dioxide (CO2)
A gaseous waste product of bodily processes that is carried by the blood to the lungs where it is exhaled.

Cardiology
The branch of medicine dealing with the heart and circulation.

Cardiopulmonary resuscitation (CPR)
A method of reviving a person whose heartbeat and breathing has stopped or slowed abnormally.

Case Manager
A patient advocate who coordinates health services and home care with the insurance company during hospitalization.

Cath toes
Temporary discoloration of a baby's toes due to decreased blood flow to the toes, sometimes due to tiny blood clots forming around an umbilical artery catheter.

Catheter
A thin tube used to administer fluids to the body or to drain fluids from the body.

CBC
See complete blood count.

Central nervous system (CNS)
The brain and spinal cord.

Central Line
A small plastic tube that is placed in a major vein of the body to deliver IVs or medications which allows the baby to avoid many needle stick if they are in long term care.

Cerclage
A surgical procedure in which the cervix is sewn shut to prevent it's opening at an early stage of pregnancy and causing a premature delivery.

Cerebral Palsy (CP)
Cerebral palsy is a term used to describe a group of chronic conditions affecting body movement and muscle coordination. It is caused by damage to one or more specific areas of the brain.

Cerebrospinal Fluid (CSF)
Fluid that circulates around the spinal column and brain.
Cervix
The lower section of the uterus, which dilates and effaces (thins and shortens) during labor and delivery to allow for the passage of the infant.

Charge nurse
The nurse in the unit who is in charge of nursing care for that shift.

Chest tube
A tube surgically inserted through the chest wall and into the chest cavity (between the collapsed lung and the chest wall) to remove air or blood that has caused a lung to collapse.

Chorioamnionitis
This is an inflammatory condition of pregnancy affecting the uterus.

Chronic lung disease (CLD)
A term used to describe long-term lung disease.

Clinical nurse specialist
The clinical nurse specialist may carry out special medical procedures, or may be involved with education of parents and staff and has received special training, through a master's degree program.

CMV (cytomegalovirus)
A virus that can cause birth defects in extremely premature babies.

CNS (central nervous system)
Refers to the brain and spinal cord.

Cochlear implant
Sometimes called a "bionic ear," the cochlear implant is a device that is surgically implanted in the inner ear; it picks up sounds from the environment and directly stimulates the auditory nerve. A cochlear implant is one approach to dealing with a profound hearing impairment.

Colostomy
A surgically created opening to allow the colon, the lower section of the large intestine, to empty directly through the abdominal wall into a bag. This is usually as a result of NEC.

Colostrum
Protein and antibody rich fluid produced in late pregnancy or in the first 3-5 days after delivery. This milk is usually yellowish in color and is especially rich in nutrients and antibodies.

Complete blood count (CBC)
A blood test to determine the number and types of cells found in blood. This test checks for cells that may be associated with infection as well as assessing for anemia.

Conductive hearing loss
Conductive hearing loss occurs when sound is not conducted efficiently through the outer ear canal to the eardrum and the tiny bones, or ossicles, of the middle ear.

Cone biopsy
A surgical procedure in which tissue from the cervix is removed to check it for malignancy. The procedure is associated with an increased risk for later preterm delivery.

Congenital Diaphragmatic Hernia (CDH)
A type of birth defect in which a hole in the diaphragm (the large muscle that separates the chest and the abdomen) allows abdominal organs to come into the chest, causing poor development of the lung on one or both sides.

Congestive heart failure (CHF)
Failure of the heart to perform efficiently because of a circulatory imbalance. This condition can occur in patent ductus arteriosus (PDA).

Continuous positive airway pressure (CPAP)
Pressurized air, usually delivery by nasal prongs or face mask, which is delivered to the baby's lungs to keep them from collapsing as the baby inhales and exhales.

Corrected age
The age of a premature baby determined by adding his postnatal days to his gestational age at birth. A baby who is fourteen days old and was born at twenty-six weeks would have a corrected age of twenty-eight weeks. 2. The age a premature baby would be if he had been born on his due date. For example, a baby born 2 months early is, at the actual age of 7 months, only 5 months old according to his corrected age.

CP
See cerebral palsy.

CPAP
See continuous positive airway pressure.

CPR
See cardiopulmonary resuscitation.

Cryotherapy
The freezing of abnormal tissue to stop its growth which is usually used in severe cases of retinopathy.

CPT (Chest Physical Therapy)
Tapping or vibrating the chest of a baby with respiratory problems to loosen mucus. This is NOT painful.

CSF
See cerebrospinal fluid.

Cultures and sensitivities
Samples of fluid or other material from the body are placed in special cultures that encourage the growth of any infectious organisms present. Organisms that grow are then tested for their sensitivity to various antibiotics.

Cyanosis
Blue or gray color of the skin caused by poor circulation or low oxygen concentration in the bloodstream.

Cytomegalovirus (CMV)
A viral infection that may infect a baby either before or after birth. In some cases CMV causes severe illness and birth defects.

D
Dc
Medical abbreviation for "discontinue," i.e. "stop"

Decadron
The trade name for dexamethasone, a steroid drug.

Developmental care
An approach to caring for premature babies that places an emphasis on their individual needs and on keeping them as free from stress as possible.

Developmental delay
A delay in reaching certain developmental milestones, relative to most other children of the same age. In preemies, developmental delays may be temporary or permanent.

Developmental Milestones
Major and minor social, emotional, physical, and cognitive skills acquired by children as they grow up.

Dexamethasone
Dexamethasone may be given to women at risk of delivering prematurely in order to promote maturation of the fetus' lungs. This has been associated with low birth weight, although not with increased rates of neonatal death.

Dextrostix
A screening blood test used to measure levels of sugar in the bloodstream at the bedside.

DIC
Abbreviation for disseminated intravascular coagulation which means no blood is clotting.

Diethylstilbestrol (DES)
A synthetic estrogen drug prescribed for pregnant women from the 1930s to the early 1970s to prevent miscarriage and premature labor. The drug was found to cause physical abnormalities in the genitalia of the daughters of women who took it. So-called DES daughters are also at increased risk of infertility, ectopic pregnancy, miscarriage, and preterm labor.

Disseminated intravascular coagulation (DIC)
A condition in which the platelets and clotting factors of the blood are consumed because of infection, hypoxia, acidosis, or other diseases or injuries. Without sufficient platelets and clotting factors, there is a tendency to bleed excessively.

Diuretic
A medication that increases the urine production to help eliminate excess body fluids.

Dizygotic twins
Fraternal twins, who don't share all of the same genes.

Donor Specific Blood
Blood that has been donated specifically for one baby from a family member or friend

Dopamine
Cardiac medicine used to improve low blood pressure.

Doppler
The monitoring device which is attached to a special blood pressure cuff to give intermittent blood pressure measurements.

Down syndrome
A chromosomal abnormality characterized by physical malformations and varying degrees of mental retardation. Often caused by an extra number 21 chromosome.

DPT (**d**iphtheria, **p**ertussis, **t**etanus)
Used to refer to the immunizations against these diseases.

Ductus arteriosus
A blood vessel in the fetus that joins the aorta with the pulmonary artery in order to divert most blood away from the fetal lungs. This blood vessel must close after birth so that blood can flow properly to the lungs to receive oxygen.

Dx

The medical abbreviation for "diagnosis".

Dyslexia

A learning disability, dyslexia means difficulty with reading.

Dysmature

An infant whose birth weight is inappropriately low for its gestational age.

Dyspnea

Shortness of breath.

E

Early Intervention Program

Planned use of physical therapy and other interventions in the first few years of a child's life to enhance the child's development.

Echocardiogram ("Echo")

A specialized ultrasound picture of the heart. Many preemies have a cardiac ultrasound if the doctor is looking for evidence of a patent ductus arteriosus.

Eclampsia

An acute and life-threatening complication of pregnancy, is characterized by the appearance of tonic-clonic seizures in a patient who had developed preeclampsia; rarely does eclampsia occur without preceding preeclamptic symptoms.

Edema
Fluid retention in the body tissues that causes puffiness or swelling. It may occur in the lungs where it can be seen on x-ray.

EEG - (electroencephalogram)
A tracing of the electrical impulses of the brain used to assess brain function and evaluate seizures.

EKG (electrocardiogram)
A tracing of the electrical pattern of the baby's heart beats.

Electrodes
Small patches taped to the baby's chest, arms or legs connected to a monitor to measure the heart and breathing rates.

Electrocardiogram (ECG or EKG)
A test that records the electrical activity of the heart. It can show abnormal rhythms (arrhythmias or dysrhythmias) or detect heart muscle damage.

Electroencephalogram (EEG)
A tracing of the electrical impulses of the brain.

Electrolytes
Chemicals that, when dissolved in water, can conduct an electrical current. The main electrolytes in the human body are sodium (Na) and Potassium (K). They play important roles in the proper functioning of the cells.

Embryo
The term used to describe the early stages of fetal growth, approximately the fourth to ninth week of pregnancy.

Endotracheal Tube (ET Tube)
A plastic tube inserted into the baby's trachea (windpipe) to assist the baby's breathing usually connected to a ventilator. You will not hear the baby cry while this tube is in place.

Enterostomy
An operation in which the surgeon makes a passage into the patient's small intestine through the abdomen with an opening in the skin of his belly during bowel surgery.

Epilepsy
A disorder of the nervous system that results in periodic convulsions or seizures

Episiotomy
An incision made to widen the vaginal opening during childbirth.

ER
Emergency room

Erythroblastosis fetalis
Erythroblastosis fetalis refers to two potentially disabling or fatal blood disorders in infants: Rh incompatibility disease and ABO incompatibility disease. Either disease may be apparent before birth and can cause fetal death in some cases. The disorder is caused by incompatibility between a mother's blood and her unborn baby's blood.

Erythrocyte
A red blood cell

Erythropoietin
A hormone produced by the kidney that promotes the formation of red blood cells in the bone marrow.

Esophagus
The tube extending from the mouth to the stomach that
carries food to the stomach.

Estriol levels
A series of tests to check the mother's blood or urine for the
hormone estriol. The tests are done to assess fetal well-
being over a period of time.

ET tube (endotracheal tube)
A flexible plastic tube that is inserted through the baby's
nose or mouth and down into the lungs. The ET tube is
hooked up to a ventilator machine.

Exchange transfusion
A type of blood transfusion in which the infant's blood is
removed in small amounts and simultaneously replaced
with the same amounts of donor blood, sometimes used to
treat severe jaundice.

Extracorporeal Membrane Oxygenation (ECMO)
This long name means "oxygenation outside the body." It's
used for babies whose lungs are not working properly
despite other treatments. The ECMO takes over the work of
the lungs so they can rest and heal. It's similar to the heart-
lung bypass used during some types of surgeries.

Extremely Low Birth Weight (ELBW)
A baby born weighing less than 2 pounds, 3 ounces (1,000
grams). Also known as a "micropreemie."

Extubate
Removing the Endotracheal Tube (ET Tube) from the
baby's windpipe.

F

Fellow
A neonatology fellow is a physician who has finished his or her residency in pediatrics and is training to become a full neonatologist. There are fellows in all specialties.

Flaring
Nasal flaring or widening of the nostrils with each breath. A sign that the baby is having minor difficulty breathing.

Fetal circulation
The special pattern of blood flow in an unborn baby in which the blood flows to and from the placenta to receive oxygen and nutrients, and to discharge wastes.

Fetal fibronectin
A protein helping to keep the placenta and membranes attached to the uterine lining. Low free levels of fibronectin detected on a swab of the vagina or cervix can help reassure that a preterm delivery is not imminent.

Fetus
The developing baby from approximately the ninth week of pregnancy until birth.

Fibroids
Benign (noncancerous) growths in the uterine wall.

Fine motor skills
Skills involving the coordination of the small muscles such as those in the hand.

Fontanel
The soft spot on the top of the baby's head.

Fraternal twins
Twins formed when two eggs are simultaneously released and fertilized.

Full-term (FT)
An infant born between the thirty-eighth and forty-second weeks of gestation.

G
GA
See gestational age.

Gastrostomy
A surgically created opening in the stomach to provide nutrition to the baby when the esophagus is blocked or injured, or to provide drainage after abdominal surgery.

Gastroesophageal reflux
Often referred to as "GE reflux" or just "reflux", this is a condition in which food in the stomach comes back up into the esophagus, and sometimes all the way out of the mouth. It is similar to heartburn in adults.

Gavage Feeding
A method of feeding breast milk or formula through a small tube passed through the baby's mouth or nose into the stomach or intestines.

Genetic abnormality
A disorder arising from abnormalities in the chromosomes of each cell that may or may not be hereditary (passed on in a family). Chromosomes are made up of "genes" which contain basic information for the growth and development of the fetus or person.

Genetic counseling
Advice and information provided by trained professional counselors on the detection and risk of occurrence of genetic disorders.

Gentamicin
A type of antibiotic used to treat many types of bacterial infection.

Gestation
The period of development from the time of fertilization of the egg, until birth. Normal gestation is 40 weeks; a premature baby is one born at or before the 37th week of pregnancy.

Gestational Age
The length of time from conception to birth. A full-term infant has a gestational age of 38-42 weeks.

Glucose
The type of sugar that circulates in the blood and is used by the body for energy.

Gram
A unit of measuring weight. 30 grams = 1 ounce. Each baby is weighed daily and the weight is measured in grams.

Gram stain
A technique in which certain types of dyes are used to stain tissue and bacteria so that they become easily visible under the microscope.

Grasping Reflex
A newborn's reflexive grab at an object, such as a finger, when it touches her hand. This grasp may be strong enough to support the infant's own weight, but doesn't last very long. This reflex lasts until a baby is 3 or 4 months old. Newborns have many naturally occurring reflexes.

Group B Streptococcus
A bacterial infection that is passed from mother to baby as they pass through the birth canal. This can be prevented in many cases by advanced screening before birth.

Grunting
A noise made by the baby indicating respiratory distress.

Guaiac
Pronounced "GWY-ak," this is a test performed on a sample of a baby's stool, to see whether there is any blood in it that isn't visible to the naked eye.

H
HA (hyperalimentation)
See total parenteral nutrition.

Head Ultrasound
A painless procedure used for looking at structures in the brain using sound waves; used in detecting bleeding into the brain or other suspected abnormalities.

Hearing Screen
Test to examine the hearing of a newborn infant.

Heart Murmur
An extra humming sound heard between beats of the heart. Innocent, functional heart murmurs are common and often heard in infants and toddlers.

Heel stick
A method of obtaining blood samples by pricking the baby's heel.

HELLP syndrome
Short for Hemolysis, Elevated Liver enzymes, and Low Platelets, HELLP syndrome is a life-threatening obstetric complication usually considered to be a variant of pre-eclampsia.

Hematocrit (Crit)
A test done to measure the concentration of red blood cells in the blood.

Hematology
The medical specialty dealing with blood disorders.

Hemoglobin (hgb., hb)
A substance in red blood cells that contains iron and carries oxygen.

Hemolysis
The rupture or breakdown of red blood cells.

Heparin Lock
A small, hollow, needle put into the hand, foot or scalp through which medicine is given intermittently.

Hernia
A weakness in the abdominal wall that causes a portion of the intestines to protrude underneath the skin around the belly button area or in the groin.

Herpes
A virus that produces sores on the mouth or genitals. An infant may become infected passing through an infected birth canal. It can cause a severe body-wide-infection often leading to death or neurological damage.

High Frequency Ventilation
A special form of mechanical ventilation, designed to help reduce complications to a preemies' delicate lungs.

High Frequency Oscillatory Ventilator
A special ventilator capable of breathing for a baby at rates exceeding those of a normal ventilator (for example, 120 - 1,320 BPM, or Breaths Per Minute).

High-risk (at-risk)
Refers to persons or situations needing special intervention to prevent illness, damage, or death, or to keep illness or damage from worsening. (i.e. high-risk newborns, high-risk pregnancies).

HMD
HMD occurs when there is not enough of a substance in the lungs called surfactant. Surfactant is made by the cells in the airways and consists of phospholipids and protein.

House officer (HO)
Intern, nurse specialist, nurse practitioner, or resident. A house officer may be the person on first call; in other words, he or she is the first person to be consulted on medical aspects of the baby's care. Some hospitals have attending physicians as the "in-house" person on call.

House staff
Another term used to refer to the house officers. Usually a doctor in residency training.

Hyaline membrane disease (HMD)
Also known as respiratory distress syndrome (RDS). Respiratory distress that affects premature babies. It is caused by a lack of surfactant, the substance that keeps the lung air sacs (alveoli) from collapsing.

Hydrocephalus
Abnormal accumulation of cerebrospinal fluid within the ventricles of the brain. It is sometimes known as "water on the brain."

Hyperactivity
See minimal brain dysfunction.

Hyperalimentation
A yellow IV solution which contains protein, sugar, and necessary vitamins and minerals given to a baby who will not be able to take full milk feedings for several days or weeks.

Hyperbilirubinemia
Another name for jaundice.

Hypercalcemia
An abnormally high amount of calcium in the blood.

Hypercapnia (hypercarbia)
An excess of carbon dioxide in the bloodstream.

Hyperglycemia
Abnormally high blood sugar levels.

Hyperkalemia
Excessive amounts of potassium in the blood.

Hypernatremia
Excessive amounts of sodium in the blood.

Hypertension
High blood pressure.
Hyperthermia
Abnormally high body temperature.

Hyperventilation
Abnormally rapid breathing.

Hypocalcemia
Abnormally low levels of calcium in the blood.

Hypoglycemia
Abnormally low blood sugar levels.

Hypokalemia
Too little potassium in the blood.

Hyponatremia
Too little sodium in the blood.

Hypotension
Abnormally low blood pressure.

Hypothermia
Abnormally low body temperature, a frequent problem with low-birth weight premature babies.

Hypovolemia
An abnormally low volume of blood in the body.

Hypoxia
A lack of sufficient oxygen.

Hysterosalpingogram
A test in which dyes, visible on an x-ray, are injected into the womb and Fallopian tubes. X-rays are then taken to detect any structural abnormalities of the reproductive organs.

I
I and O
Abbreviation for "input and output." It refers to the amount of fluids given by oral feedings or by IV, and the amount of fluid excreted in the urine or stools, as well as blood removed for testing, over a given period of time.

Iatrogenic
An injury or disease caused by medical treatment.

ICH
See intracranial hemorrhage.

ICN
Abbreviation for "intensive care nursery".

Identical twins
Twins that result from the accidental division of a single
fertilized egg.

IDEA
An acronym for the Individuals with Disabilities Education
Act, which provides grants to states to support services,
including evaluation and assessment, for young children
who have or are at risk of developmental delays/
disabilities. Birth To Three is a program under IDEA.

Idiopathic
Something which happens spontaneously or from an
unknown cause.

IL
See intralipid.

Ileostomy
A surgically created opening to allow the ileus, the part of
the intestine above the colon, to empty directly through the
abdominal wall.

IM
See intramuscular injection.

Ileal Perforation
Puncture or hole in the last part of the small bowel (ileum).
This usually occurs spontaneously in extremely premature
babies. Its cause is unknown. Often an ileal perforation
requires surgery to form an ileostomy and to repair the hole
in the bowel. Some NICUs have reported success simply by
putting a piece of drainage tubing into the abdomen to drain
out the infection and let the perforation seal on its own.

Inborn
A child born and treated in the same hospital, a baby who was not transported to receive intensive care.

Incompetent cervix
A cervix that opens in mid to late pregnancy, often causing a miscarriage or premature birth.

Individualized Family Service Plan (IFSP)
A written statement for an infant or toddler developed by a team of people who have worked with the child and the family. The IFSP describes the child's development levels, family information, major outcomes expected to be achieved for the child and family, the services the child will be receiving, when and where the child will receive these services, and the steps to be taken to support the transition of the child to another program.

Incubator
A clear plastic box which keeps babies warm and protects them from germs and noise.

Indomethacin
An aspirin-like drug sometimes used to close the patent ductus arteriosus.

Informed consent
Permission that a person or the guardian of a patient gives for a specific medical procedure after the risks, benefits, and alternatives have been fully explained by the physician.

Infusion pump
A pump attached to an intravenous line to deliver IV fluids to the baby in tiny, precisely measured amounts.

Intern
A doctor just out of medical school.

Intracranial Hemorrhage
Bleeding within the skull. Bleeding most often occurs
within the ventricles of premature infants, but it can occur
anywhere within or on the outside of the brain.

Intralipid
A white IV solution containing a high concentration of fat
(lipid).

Intramuscular injection (IM)
An injection into the muscle; in a premature baby,
injections are usually given into the thigh muscle.

Intrauterine growth retardation (IUGR)
A term that is used to describe a baby that grows
abnormally slow while in the womb.

Intravenous (IV)
A small plastic tube placed directly through the skin into
the vein so nutrients, fluids and medications can flow into
the baby.

Intraventricular Hemorrhage (IVH)
Bleeding into the ventricles (fluid-filled spaces) of the
brain.

Intubation
The insertion of a tube into the trachea (windpipe) to allow
air to reach the lungs which assists with breathing.

In utero
Within the womb.

Isolette
Also known as an incubator, an isolette is a clear plastic, enclosed bassinet used to keep prematurely born infants warm.

IUGR (intrauterine growth retardation)
A term that is used to describe a baby that grows abnormally slow while in the womb.

IV (Intravenous) Fluids
A small plastic tube placed directly through the skin into the vein so nutrients, fluids and medications can flow into the baby.

IVC
Indwelling venous catheter.

IVH (intraventricular hemorrhage)
Bleeding occurring in an inner part of the brain, near the ventricles, where premature babies have blood vessels that are particularly fragile and prone to rupture.

J
Jaundice
Jaundice comes from the accumulation of a natural waste product, bilirubin., causing yellowing of the skin and eyes.
Jugular veins
Large veins on either side of the neck that return blood to the heart from the head and neck.

K
K
Chemical symbol for potassium.

Kangaroo Care
Skin-to-skin contact between parent and baby. During kangaroo care, the baby is placed on the parent's chest, dressed only in a diaper. The baby's head is turned to the side so the baby can hear the parent's heartbeat and feel the parent's warmth. Kangaroo care is extremely effective if the baby is stable.

Kernicterus
A form of brain damage caused by excessive jaundice.

Kilogram (kg)
Unit of weight of the metric system that equals 1000 grams or 2.2 pounds.

L
Lab Tech
A person from the laboratory who draws blood samples for the tests ordered by doctors.

Labor
Process by which the cervix shortens (effaces) and opens (dilates) to allow the baby to pass from the womb into the world.

Lactation
Production of milk by the breasts for your infant.

Lactation Consultant
A person within the hospital who is trained to assist mothers with breast pumping or breastfeeding.

Lactose
Sugar found in human milk.

Lanugo
Soft and fuzzy hair which some premature babies are born with.It disappears as the baby matures.

Large for gestational age (LGA)
Newborn infant who is above the 90th percentile in weight at birth for his gestational age.

Large motor skills
Skills such as walking or crawling that involve the coordination of large muscle groups.

Laryngoscope
Tool with a long, lighted, hollow metal tube and handle. Used in intubation to see the vocal cords and guide the tube between them.

Lasix
A diuretic.

LBW
See low birth weight infant.

Lead Wires
The wires connecting the sensors on the baby's chest to the vital signs monitor.

Let-down reflex
Release of milk into the milk ducts and down to the nipple.

Leukocyte (white blood cell)
A type of blood cell that protects the body against harmful substances such as bacteria and viruses.

Level
A marker of the level of infant care a NICU can provide, usually expressed as I, IIa/IIb, or IIIa/IIIb/IIIc.

LGA
See large for gestational age.

Low birth weight infant (LBW) - baby who weighs less than 5 ½ pounds (2500 gm) at birth; can be premature or full-term.

Lower respiratory tract infection (LRI)
 An infection affecting the larynx (voice box), trachea (wind-pipe), bronchial tubes, the bronchioles, or the lungs.

LP
An abbreviation for a lumbar puncture.

LPN
An abbreviation for Licensed Practical Nurse.

L/S ratio
The ratio between lecithin and sphingomyelin (components of surfactant) in the amniotic fluid. The ratio indicates the maturity of the unborn baby's lungs.

Lumbar Puncture (LP)
A test that involves inserting a hollow needle in between the vertebrae of the lower back to collect a sample of cerebrospinal fluid.

LVN
Licensed vocational nurse.

Low Birth Weight (LBW)
A baby born weighing less than 5 1/2 pounds (2,500 grams) and more than 3 pounds, 5 ounces (1,500 grams) — see Very Low Birth Weight.

M
Magnesium sulfate
A drug used in the treatment of toxemia and in stopping pre-term labor.

Magnetic Resonance Imaging (MRI)
An imaging technique that uses powerful magnets and computers to produce a detailed picture of body tissue.

Mastitis
An inflammation of the mammary gland in the breast.

Meconium
A dark green, sticky mucus, (a mixture of amniotic fluid and secretions from the intestinal glands), normally found in infants' intestines. It is the first stool passed by the newborn. Passage of meconium within the uterus before birth can be a sign of fetal distress.

Meconium Aspiration Syndrome (MAS)
Breathing problems that occur when babies inhale meconium or meconium-stained amniotic fluid into their lungs.

Meconium staining
Refers to staining of the amniotic fluid, placenta, infant's umbilical cord, skin or nails with meconium. In some instances, meconium stained fluid indicates the fetus was in distress before birth.

Meningitis
Inflammation or infection of the meninges, the membranes surrounding the brain and spinal cord.

Meningocele
A birth defect in which there is a protrusion of the meninges (the tissue lining the brain and spinal cord) through an opening in the skull or spinal column.

Mental retardation
Limited intellectual development.

Metabolism
All the life-sustaining processes carried out by the cells in the body.

Monitor
Machine that displays and often records the heart rate, respiratory rate, blood pressure and blood oxygen saturation of the baby. An alarm may sound if one or a number of these vital signs are abnormal.

Monozygotic twins
Identical twins that have the same genes.

Moro Reflex
Often called a startle reflex because it usually occurs when a baby is startled by a loud sound or movement. In response to the sound, the baby throws back his/her head, extends out the arms and legs, cries, then pulls the arms and legs back in.

Motor Skills
Gross motor skills are the movements that use the large muscles in the arms, legs, and torso, such as running and jumping. Fine motor skills are the small muscle movements used to grasp and manipulate objects, like picking up a raisin.

Mucus
A sticky secretion produced by mucous membranes such as the nose and throat.

Multidisciplinary
Many different areas of expertise or specialization coming together to provide comprehensive care. (Examples include medicine, nursing, pharmacy, social work, physical therapy and respiratory therapy.)

Murmur (Heart Murmur)
An extra heart sound that is heard when listening to the baby's heart with a stethoscope; this may be normal or abnormal.

Myopia
Nearsightedness.

N
Na
A chemical symbol for sodium.

Narcotic
A type of drug that relieves pain and produces sleep.

Nasal cannula
A set of plastic prongs and tubing that delivers extra oxygen into a baby's nose.

Nasal CPAP
Continuous positive airway pressure administered to an
infant through nasal prongs.

Naso-gastric tube (NG tube)
A small plastic tube inserted through the nose or mouth and
into the stomach. This tube is used for gavage feedings
when an infant is unable to bottle or direct breastfeed.
NBICU
An abbreviation for newborn intensive care unit.

Nebulizer
A device that is used to give the baby inhaled medications.

Necrotizing enterocolitis (NEC)
An intestinal infection, most common in young preemies,
in which portions of the bowel are damaged or destroyed
because of poor blood flow, inflammation, or infection.

Neonatal nurse practitioner (NNP)
A registered nurse who has received additional training,
usually through a master's degree program, and who is
qualified to provide certain aspects of the baby's medical
care under the supervision of a physician.

Neonatal period
The first 30 days of life.

Neonatal Pharmacist
A person who is specially trained and educated in
dispensing medication for babies.

Neonate
A term used to describe an infant during the first 30 days of
life.

Neonatal Intensive Care Unit (NICU)
A special care nursery for preemies and newborn infants with severe medical complications. They are cared for by neonatologists and nurses with specialty training.

Neonatologist
A pediatrician who has received 4-6 years of advanced training after medical school in preparation for treating premature or sick newborns. This is the person who usually directs your baby's care if hospitalization in an NICU is required.

Neurologist
A physician who specializes in the conditions of the brain and nervous system.

Newborn intensive care unit (NICU NBISU, NBIC, ICN)
Section of a hospital with trained staff and special equipment to care for critically ill newborns. See *NICU*

NG Tube
See Nasogastric tube.

NICU
Short for **Neonatal Intensive Care Unit**. An NICU is a hospital unit where preemies that require complex medical care are taken care of, along with other critically ill or medical unstable newborns.

Nippling
Sucking on a bottle filled with formula or breast-milk.

NNP
See Neonatal Nurse Practitioner.

Non-stress test
A test in which the unborn baby's heartbeat is monitored to detect abnormal patterns indicating fetal distress.

NPO
An abbreviation for a Latin term that means "nothing by mouth" -- i.e., no food or water.

Nurse
A person specially trained to care for the sick. NICU nurses are specially trained to care for premature and sick infants and their families.

O

OB
The abbreviation for "obstetrician".

Obstructive apnea
A pause in breathing that occurs because a baby's airway is obstructed and little air can get through. This can happen even when a baby is moving his chest to breathe.

Occupational/Physical Therapist
A person who evaluates your baby's neurologic (brain) development and plans exercises to help development, improve muscle control and solve feeding problems.

O2 Sat
Oxygen saturation. The level of oxygen in the baby's bloodstream. Nurses say the baby's "sats are stable".

Oligohydramnois
A condition of too little amniotic fluid.

Omphalocele
A birth defect in which the intestines (and sometimes other abdominal organs such as the liver) push against the base of the umbilical cord.

"on-call"
Physician or nurse specialist who can be summoned at a particular time to make and carry out medical decisions in the nursery.

Ophthalmologist
A physician specializing in diseases of the eye.

OR
Abbreviation for operating room.

Orthopedist
A physician specializing in diseases of the bone.

Oscillating ventilator
Also called a high-frequency ventilator, it works differently than a conventional ventilator. An oscillating ventilator keeps a baby's lungs continuously inflated by providing tiny quantities of air at extremely rapid rates.

Osteopenia of Prematurity (OOP)
A decrease in the amount of calcium and phosphorus in the bones. This can cause bones to be weak and brittle, and increases the risk for broken bones.

OT
Abbreviation for occupational therapist.

Otitis media
A bacterial or viral infection of the middle ear.

Otolaryngologist
A physician specializing in disease of the ears, nose, and throat.

Otologist
A physician who specializes in disorders of the ear.

Outborn
A baby who is transported after birth to a tertiary care center for treatment.

Oximeter (Pulse Oximeter)
Machine monitoring the amount of oxygen in the blood. A tape-like cuff is wrapped around the baby's toe, foot, hand or finger. This machine allows the NICU staff to monitor the amount of oxygen in the baby's blood without having to obtain blood for laboratory testing.

Oxygen (O2)
The gas that makes up 21% of the atmosphere. The amount of oxygen delivered to an infant can be controlled from 21% to 100%.

Oxygen Hood (Oxyhood)
A clear plastic hood placed over the baby's head to give him a measured amount of oxygen.

Oxytocin - (Pitocin)
A hormone that stimulates uterine contractions and the "let-down response" in lactating mothers.

P

Parenteral Nutrition (Hyperalimentation)
Solution put directly into the bloodstream, giving necessary nutrients, such as protein, carbohydrates, vitamins, minerals, salts, and fat.

Patent Ductus Arteriosus (PDA)
A heart problem that is seen in premature babies. A PDA may be treated either with medication or surgery.

Pavulon (pancuronium)
A drug that produces temporary paralysis. It may be used to keep a baby from fighting the respirator.

p.c.
The abbreviation for the Latin words meaning "after a meal."

pCO$_2$
The partial pressure of arterial carbon dioxide; a measure of the carbon dioxide content of the blood.

PDA (patent ductus arteriosus)
A heart condition in which an extra fetal blood vessel next to the heart remains open after birth instead of closing as it should.

PDBM/PDHM
Abbreviations for pasteurized donor breast milk/ pasteurized donor human milk. Milk from donor mothers that is heat treated and therefore sterile. It is used when a mother is unable to produce enough breast milk for her infant.

Pediatrician
A doctor who specializes in the care of infants and children.

Perinatal
The perinatal period commences at 22 completed weeks and ends seven completed days after birth.

Perinatologist
A physician who has completed training in obstetrics and takes further training in the care of high-risk pregnancies.

Periodic breathing
Rapid breaths followed by long pauses which is a normal breathing pattern among preemies.

Peripheral IVs
An IV usually in the baby's arms, legs or scalp that only extends into the vein a short distance.

Periventricular Leukomalacia (PVL)
Damage to part of the brain caused by complications of prematurity. The brain tissue that has been lost is important to the control of muscle movements in the legs and sometimes in the arms. PVL is often associated with cerebral palsy and other developmental problems.

Persistent fetal circulation (PFC)
A newborn baby's circulation changes back to the circulation of a fetus, where much of the blood flow bypasses the lungs.

Persistent Pulmonary Hypertension of the Newborn (PPHN)
High blood pressure in the lungs, which causes breathing problems and reduced levels of oxygen in the blood.

Petechiae
Pinpoint-sized red dots under the surface of the skin.

pH
It expresses the degree to which a solution is acid or alkaline. The lower the pH, the more acid is present.

Phenobarbital
A drug used to control seizures.

Phototherapy
A treatment for jaundice by placing a blue fluorescent light over the baby's bed to help break down bilirubin into a water-soluble form that can be eliminated in the kidneys.

Physical therapist (PT)
A therapist who treats problems of coordination and of the large motor skills.

PICC Line
A special IV line used to provide fluids into a vein. A PICC line is usually very stable and lasts longer than a typical IV.

PIE (pulmonary interstitial emphysema)
A condition occurring in infants on ventilators that results in the formation of "bubbles" around the tiny air sacs (the alveoli) of the lungs. These "bubbles" may interfere with normal lung function.

Placental abruption/abruptio
A pregnancy complication, usually (but not always) signaled by vaginal bleeding and abdominal pain, in which part of the placenta detaches from the wall of the uterus, affecting the blood and oxygen supply to the fetus.

Placenta previa
Condition where the **placenta** lies low in the uterus and partially or completely covers the cervix.

Plasma
Clear, fluid portion of blood (after the red blood cells have been removed).

Platelets
A blood cell that is needed for proper clotting; also called thrombocytes.

Pneumogram (sleep study) or Pneumocardiogram (PCG)
A painless study of an infant's heart and respiratory patterns done over a continuous 12-hour period to detect any abnormal breathing patterns. It is used to evaluate apnea.

Pneumonia
An inflammation or infection of the lungs.

Pneumothorax
When air from the baby's lungs leaks out into the space between the baby's lungs and chest wall. While small leaks may require no treatment, larger leaks may cause serious complications such as lung collapse and may need to be repaired with surgery.

PO_2 (PaO_2)
The partial pressure of arterial carbon dioxide; a measure of the carbon dioxide content of the blood.

Polycythemia
An abnormally high number of red blood cells, a condition that causes "sluggish" circulation. In babies, it can cause breathing difficulties, low blood sugar, and jaundice.

Polyhydramnios
An excessive amount of amniotic fluid, which can overly distend the uterus, and lead to preterm labor and delivery.

Positive end expiratory pressure (PEEP)
On a respirator, the constant amount of pressure exerted on the infant's lungs to keep them expanded during and after breaths.

Postpartum
After delivery.

Postural drainage (PD)
A method of tilting the baby in various positions to allow mucus to drain easily from his lungs.

Preeclampsia
A medical term to define the maternal condition of elevated blood pressure, edema of the hands and feet, and the presence of protein in the urine during a woman's pregnancy.

Pregnancy-induced hypertension (PIH)
See preeclampsia.

Premature infant
An infant who is less than thirty-seven completed weeks' gestational age at birth.

Premature rupture of the membranes (PROM)
The breaking of the membranes surrounding the fetus before the beginning of labor; may occur before a term or a preterm delivery.
Prenatal
Before birth.

Progesterone
A hormone of pregnancy thought to protect the developing fetus.

Projectile vomiting
Extremely forceful ejection of the stomach contents.

Prostaglandins
Substances found in body tissues that can cause contractions of the smooth muscles and the widening of certain blood vessels. Prostaglandins are thought to be involved in the process of labor.

Pseudomonas
A type of bacteria.

PT
An abbreviation for physical therapist.

Pulmonary hypertension
An inability of the blood vessels of the lungs to relax and open up normally after birth. Poor circulation through the lungs and poor oxygenation of the blood result. Respiratory therapy and inhaled or IV drugs may be used to relax the lungs' constricted vessels to help treat this condition.

Pulmonary insufficiency of the premature (PIP)
A type of respiratory distress afflicting the youngest premature infants. It is caused as much by an immaturity of the lung tissue as by a lack of surfactant. The treatment is the same as for RDS.

Pulmonary Interstitial Emphysema (PIE)
A condition occurring in infants on ventilators that results in the formation of "bubbles" around the tiny air sacs (the alveoli) of the lungs. These "bubbles" may interfere with normal lung function.

Pulse oximeter
A monitoring device used to determine blood oxygen levels. This noninvasive device is taped to the skin, usually a finger or foot, for oxygen level readings.

PVL (see periventricular leukomalacia)
Cysts in the white matter of the brain near the ventricles, indicating areas that have been permanently damaged. It is the most common ischemic brain injury in premature infants.

Q
q
Medical abbreviation for "every."

q.d.
Medical abbreviation for "every day."

q.h.
Medical abbreviation for "every hour."

q.i.d.
Medical abbreviation for "four times a day."

q.o.d.
Medical abbreviation for "every other day."

q.s.
Medical abbreviation for "a sufficient amount."

q.wk.
Medical abbreviation for "every week."

R
Radiant warmer
An open-air bed with overhead heating above it. This type of bed is used in the NICU immediately after delivery to allow easy access to the baby and also to help maintain a baby's body temperature.

Radiology (X-ray) Tech
A person who is trained in taking x-rays.

Rales
Abnormal crackling noises in the chest made by air passing through congested bronchial tubes.

RBC
Red blood cell

RDS (respiratory distress syndrome)
A serious breathing problem which is the result of a preemie having immature lungs.

Red blood cells (RBC)
RBCs are a part of the body's blood that contains hemoglobin and carries oxygen to all the cells and tissues of the body.

Regionalization
A system for providing appropriate care to all mothers and infants within a specific geographical region.
Perinatal care may be provided at primary (Level I) , secondary (Level II), or tertiary (Level III or IV) centers depending on the risk status of mother and baby.

Resident
A doctor in his or her specialty training years.

Residuals
The amount of undigested food left in the stomach after a reasonable length of time has elapsed for digestion.

Respirator
A mechanical device used to substitute for, or to assist with breathing.

Respiratory Distress Syndrome (RDS)
See RDS

Respiratory Syncytial Virus (RSV)
RSV infection is a particular risk for infants with chronic lung problems and those born prematurely. In adults the virus causes cold like symptoms but in premature babies it may lead to pneumonia. The RSV season is usually from October to March.

Retina
The lining of the back of the eye that receives visual images and relays messages to the brain.

Retinopathy of Prematurity (ROP)
Abnormal growth of the blood vessels in the retina, the layer of cells in the back of the eye. The retina does not mature until close to term (40 weeks gestation), so when babies are born very prematurely, the normal growth of blood vessels into the retina is altered.

Retraction
A sunken appearance of the chest wall as the baby breathes. The baby is working harder to breathe than normal.

Retrolental fibroplasia (RLF)
An eye disease of premature infants.

Rh disease
A blood incompatibility between the mother and her baby that causes the destruction of the red blood cells.

RhoGAM shots
Injections given a mother with Rh-negative blood after the birth of an Rh-positive baby. This injection prevents the mother from developing antibodies that could harm a future Rh-positive baby.

Ritodrine (Yutopar)
One of the betamimetic drugs used to stop preterm labor.

RLF
Abbreviation for retrolental fibroplasias.

Room Air
The air we normally breathe, which contains 21% oxygen. When supplemental oxygen is given for respiratory problems, it is in concentrations higher than 21%.

ROP
Abbreviation for retinopathy of prematurity.

RSV (respiratory syncytial virus)
A common virus that gives most people a cold, but can be more serious in premature babies, causing infections such as pneumonia or bronchiolitis.

Rooting Reflex
An instinctive reflex in newborn infants that causes them to turn their head to the side when their cheek is stroked. This reflex helps infants learn how to eat.

Rubella
A virus that causes German measles and severe intrauterine infections.

Rx
The medical abbreviation for "prescription."

S
Sats
A term for blood oxygen saturation.

Scalp IV
An intravenous needle placed in a vein in the infant's scalp.

Scleral buckle
The most common way to treat retinal detachment

Seizure
A "short-circuiting" of electrical impulses in the brain, resulting from a variety of causes.

Sensorineural hearing loss - a hearing impairment resulting from damage to the structures of the inner ear or to the nerves that conduct sound impulses to the brain.

Sepsis
A potentially dangerous infection of the bloodstream which occurs when the body's normal reaction to inflammation or a bacterial infection goes into overdrive.

Septic or Sepsis work-up
A series of tests to check for the presence of infection.

Serous otitis
Fluid accumulation in the middle ear.

SGA
See small for gestational age.

Shunt - 1. an artificially created passage between two areas of the body, a tube that drains fluid from the ventricles of the brain into the peritoneum (the abdominal cavity). .

SIDS (sudden infant death syndrome)
Crib death, the death of an infant during sleep from unknown causes.

Skin Temperature Probe
A small soft wire taped to the baby's skin to which allows the body temperature to be taken.

Sleep study
See pneumogram.

Small for gestational age (SGA) - a newborn is considered small-for-gestational age if her birth weight is below the tenth percentile on the standard growth curve for her age.

Social Worker
Some social workers act as counselors for parents undergoing personal or family stress while their baby in a NICU.

Sonogram
A picture produced by ultrasound.

Spastic diplegia - the most common type of cerebral palsy among preemies, it is characterized by stiff ("spastic") muscle tone, affecting mainly the legs and feet ("diplegia").

Special care nursery
See step-down unit.

Speech and language pathologist
A specialist in the treatment of speech problems.

Spinal tap
See lumbar puncture.

Step-down unit
May also be called an intermediate care nursery, a level II unit, or a special care nursery unit for babies that have graduated from the NICU.

Strabismus
An abnormal alignment of one or both eyes. It may cause the eyes to turn inward (crossed eyes or esotropia) or turn outward (wall eye or exotropia).

Stress test
A test to monitor fetal heart rate changes in response to induced contractions. Abnormal heart rate patterns may indicate fetal distress.

Subarachnoid hemorrhage
Bleeding in the subarachnoid space, the area around the outside of the brain.

Suction
A procedure to remove mucus and secretions from the lungs or stomach.

Sudden infant death syndrome
See SIDS

Surfactant
Surfactant is a soapy material inside the lungs of adults and mature infants that helps the lung to function without collapsing. Lung surfactant production is one of the last systems to mature in an infant, which can cause the breathing problems found in preemies.
The use of surfactant to treat respiratory problems in preemies is one of the most important recent medical advances in pediatrics.

Swaddling
Securely wrapping a baby in a light blanket as a soothing device.

Symmetric growth restriction
When an SGA, or small-for-gestational-age baby, has a head circumference, length and birth weight, that are below the tenth percentile for her age.

Synchronized Intermittent Mandatory Ventilation (SIMV)
The ventilator mode where the mechanical breaths given by the ventilator are synchronized with the baby's spontaneous (regular) breaths

T
Tachycardia
An abnormally fast or rapid heart rate.

Tachypnea
A respiratory rate above what is considered normal for infants (above 60 breaths per minute).

Terbutaline (Brethine)
A tocolytic medication used to stop preterm labor.

Term infant
An infant born between approximately thirty-eight and forty-two weeks of gestation.

Tertiary center
See regionalization.

Theophylline
A medication used to stimulate breathing. It is prescribed to reduce the incidence of apneic episodes.

Thermoregulation
A regulation of body temperature.

Thrombocytes
Cells that play a key role in blood clotting.

Thrombocytopenia
Is a condition in which there is a deficient number of circulating platelets.

Thrush
A fungus infection of the mouth characterized by white patches on a red inflamed surface.

t.i.d.
The medical abbreviation for the Latin words meaning "three times a day."

Tocolytic drugs
Drugs used to relax the uterus and halt uterine contractions. They can be given to a pregnant woman to treat preterm labor.

Tonic Neck Reflex
When a baby's head is turned to one side, the arm on that side stretches out and the opposite arm bends up at the elbow. This is often called the "fencing" position. The tonic neck reflex lasts about six to seven months.

TORCH
A group of maternal infections that can cause serious effects on the fetus: Toxyplasmosis, Other viruses, Rubella, Cytomegalovirus, and Herpes simplex virus.

Toxemia of pregnancy
See preeclampsia.

Toxoplasmosis
A parasite infection that causes serious newborn illnesses.

TPR
Medical abbreviation for temperature, pulse, respiration.

Trachea
Windpipe; an ET tube used for mechanical ventilation that extends down into the trachea.

Tracheostomy ("Trach")
A surgical opening in the trachea, below the larynx (voice box), made to allow air to enter the lungs when the throat becomes obstructed.

Transcutaneous monitor (TCM)
Monitoring device placed on the infant's skin that records blood oxygen or carbon dioxide levels.

Trimester
A period of three months. A 9-month pregnancy is divided into first, second, and third trimesters.

TTN (Transient Tachypnea of the Newborn)
A respiratory problem seen in the newborn shortly after delivery. It consists of a period of rapid breathing (higher than the normal range of 40-60 times per minute). It is likely due to retained lung fluid, and common in 35+ week gestation babies who are delivered by caesarian section without labor.

Tube feeding
See gavage feeding.

Twin-to-twin transfusion syndrome (TTTS)
Occurs almost exclusively in a monochorionic twin gestation, involves the slow and continuous donation of blood from one fetus into the other.

U

UAC/UVC (Umbilical Artery Catheter/Umbilical Vein Catheter)
A soft plastic tube inserted into an artery or vein in the baby's naval in order to give IV fluids or medications, to monitor blood pressure and obtain blood for tests.

UAL
Umbilical artery line. See UAC/UVC.

Ultrasound (sonogram)
A diagnostic imaging technique where echoes of high frequency sound waves produce a picture of body tissues.

Umbilical Arterial Catheter (UAC)
A small tube or catheter placed in a belly button artery. It is used to check blood pressure, draw blood samples and give fluids.

Umbilical Venous Catheter (UVC)
Catheter (small tube) placed in the belly button vein. It is used to give the baby fluids and medications.

Umbilical cord
The connection between the baby and the placenta.

Upper respiratory infections (URI)
A cold; an infection affecting any portion of the respiratory tract above the larynx (voice box).

UTI
Abbreviation for urinary tract infection; usually refers to infections of the bladder.

V

Vein

A blood vessel leading to the heart.

Ventilator ("Vent")

A machine that assists in breathing. Lung immaturity in prematurely born infants is the most common reason for a newborn to require a ventilator.

Ventricle

A small chamber, as in the ventricles of the heart or brain.

Ventriculoperitoneal Shunt

A surgery performed to relieve pressure inside the skull (intracranial pressure) caused by water on the brain.

Vernix

White, fatty substance that protects the fetus' skin in the womb.

Very Low Birth Weight (VLBW)

A baby born weighing less than 3 pounds, 5 ounces (1,500 grams) and more than 2 pounds, 3 ounces (1,000 grams). See also Low Birth Weight and Extremely Low Birth Weight.

Virus

A tiny infectious organism that is unable to live on its own but thrives inside body cells.

Vision therapist

A therapist who helps visually impaired people make full use of their remaining sight.

Vitrectomy
This surgical procedure, used to repair a detached retina, removes vitreous gel from the middle of the eye so the surgeon can reach and reposition the detached portion of the retina.

Vital Signs
Measurement of the baby's temperature, heart rate, respiratory rate and blood pressure.

Vital Signs Monitor
A machine measuring and displaying heart rate, breathing rate, and blood pressure on a computer screen. If these vital signs become abnormal, an alarm usually sounds.

VP (ventriculoperitoneal) shunt
A surgery performed to relieve pressure inside the skull (intracranial pressure) caused by water on the brain

W
Ward Clerk
The nursery secretary who answers the phone and helps coordinate all the baby's records.

Warmer
Also known as a **Radiant Warmer**, this bed allows maximum access to a sick baby.

WBC
Abbreviation for white blood cell. .

Wean
To slowly decrease and then stop an intervention.

Wheeze
Whistling, humming, or raspy sound made during
breathing, caused by obstructions in the respiratory tract.

White blood cells (WBCs)
WBCs are the part of the body's blood responsible for
fighting against infection. See leukocyte.

Thank you for your time in reading
Mitchell's Gift.

www.ingramcontent.com/pod-product-compliance
Lightning Source LLC
Chambersburg PA
CBHW021158010426
R18062100001B/R180621PG41931CBX00023B/41